# Clinician's Guide to Applying, Conducting, and Disseminating Clinical Education Research

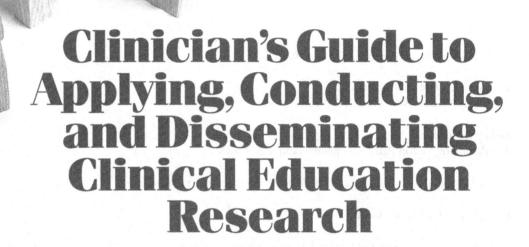

# Clinician's Guide to Applying, Conducting, and Disseminating Clinical Education Research

## Editors

### Mark DeRuiter, MBA, PhD, CCC-A/SLP, F-ASHA

Professor and Vice Chair for Academic Affairs
Clinical Science Doctoral Program
Department of Communication Science and Disorders
University of Pittsburgh
Pittsburgh, Pennsylvania

### Sarah M. Ginsberg, EdD, CCC-SLP, F-ASHA

Professor
Department of Special Education & Communication Sciences and Disorders
Eastern Michigan University
Ypsilanti, Michigan

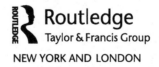

Routledge
Taylor & Francis Group

NEW YORK AND LONDON

Cover Artist: Tinhouse Design

First published in 2024 by SLACK Incorporated

Published in 2024 by Routledge
605 Third Avenue, New York, NY 10158

and by Routledge
4 Park Square, Milton Park, Abingdon, Oxon, OX14 4RN

*Routledge is an imprint of the Taylor & Francis Group, an informa business*

© 2024 Taylor & Francis Group

Library of Congress Control Number: 2023029196

ISBN: 9781638220428 (pbk)
ISBN: 9781003523192 (ebk)

DOI: 10.4324/9781003523192

# DEDICATION

To our moms, Alice DeRuiter and Marcia Ginsberg, who got us as far as they could.
To our spouses, Cathy DeRuiter and Jeff More, who couldn't get us any further but kept us anyway.

# Contents

# ACKNOWLEDGMENTS

We would like to thank our trusted colleagues in allied health fields that consulted with us about how concepts apply in their clinical fields:

Sarah L. Bolander, DMDc, PA-C, DFAAPA
Midwestern University
Glendale, Arizona

Amber Herrick, PA-C, MS
Midwestern University
Downers Grove, Illinois

Sharon Ingersoll, PharmD
Nebraska Methodist College
Omaha, Nebraska

Alice Kindschuh
Nebraska Methodist College
Omaha, Nebraska

Kristina Rask
Sullivan, Nolan, and Associates
Ann Arbor, Michigan

# ABOUT THE EDITORS

*Mark DeRuiter, MBA, PhD, CCC-A/SLP, F-ASHA* is dually certified as a speech-language pathologist and audiologist by the American Speech-Language-Hearing Association. Clinically, he has worked in a busy ear, nose, and throat practice; the hearing aid industry; schools; and private clinics. He transitioned to working in higher education in 2002 after earning his PhD from the University of Minnesota, Twin Cities. He has spent most of his higher education career at the intersection of clinical education, classroom teaching, and research. Currently, Dr. DeRuiter serves as the Director of the Clinical Science Doctorate in Speech-Language Pathology at the University of Pittsburgh and teaches across undergraduate and graduate programs in communication science and disorders. Service has been a rewarding part of his career, and he has served in a variety of roles with the American Speech-Language-Hearing Association and the Council of Academic Programs in Communication Sciences and Disorders. Throughout his career, Dr. DeRuiter has seen the need to encourage and inspire clinical educators to conduct research in the clinical education process. He is a co-author of *Basic Audiometry Learning Manual, Third Edition* and co-editor/author of *Professional Issues in Speech-Language Pathology and Audiology, Fifth Edition*.

*Sarah M. Ginsberg, EdD, CCC-SLP, F-ASHA* is an American Speech-Language-Hearing Association–certified speech-language pathologist and professor of communication sciences and disorders at Eastern Michigan University. She began working with students providing clinical education in the hospitals where she worked and then transitioned to teaching university courses and serving as a clinical educator at the university, before becoming a full-time faculty member. In her role as founding editor for *Teaching and Learning in Communication Sciences & Disorders*, she recognized that clinical educators were interested in engaging with clinical education research and wanted to provide a pathway to help them be successful with this work. She has also edited or co-authored/edited *Scholarship of Teaching and Learning in Speech-Language Pathology and Audiology: Evidence-Based Education, Xerostomia: An Interdisciplinary Approach to Managing Dry Mouth, Evidence-Based Education in the Classroom: Examples From Clinical Disciplines*, and *Simulation-Based Learning in Communication Sciences and Disorders: Moving From Theory to Practice*, the last three published by SLACK Incorporated. Her research focus has been primarily on issues of teaching and learning in clinical fields.

# Contributing Authors

*Jessica Brown, PhD, CCC-SLP (Chapter 6)*
Speech-Language Pathologist
Related/Supplemental Services
Olentangy Local School District
Powell, Ohio

*Jordan Dann, MA, CCC-SLP (Chapter 8)*
Speech Therapist
E. B. Pediatric Resources
Chicago, Illinois

*Carol C. Dudding, PhD, CCC-SLP, F-ASHA (Chapter 3)*
Professor
Communication Sciences and Disorders Department
James Madison University
Harrisonburg, Virginia

*Lizbeth H. Finestack, PhD, CCC-SLP (Chapter 5)*
Professor
Department of Speech-Language-Hearing Sciences
University of Minnesota—Twin Cities
Minneapolis, Minnesota

*Elizabeth A. VandeWaa, PhD (Chapter 11)*
Professor
Adult Health Nursing
University of South Alabama
Mobile, Alabama

*Patrick R. Walden, PhD, CCC-SLP (Chapter 7)*
Associate Professor and Chair
Department of Speech-Language Pathology
Monmouth University
West Long Branch, New Jersey

*Jayne Yatczak, PhD, OTRL (Chapter 9)*
Associate Professor of Occupational Therapy
School of Health Sciences
Eastern Michigan University
Ypsilanti, Michigan

# INTRODUCTION

Welcome! We're glad you're here. That might sound a little strange for a workbook introduction, but we believe the tone of this introduction will fit very well once you engage with what you find in the coming pages. What you're about to read is a workbook that is written by experts in the clinical education and research space. Our goal is to nurture clinicians who wish to engage in clinical education research with comfortable, digestible language. We want to leave you inspired and with a plan to engage with clinical education research, whether or not you have a "research degree."

Rather than give you outlines of all the chapters, we want you to envision a funnel. On the wide end of that funnel, we'll discuss issues related to you, your roles, and research in general. Those areas will be covered in Chapters 1 through 4. We'll then narrow things down in Chapters 5 through 8, where you'll receive advice on seeking help, formulating and refining your questions, and designing your research. Finally, Chapters 9 through 12 will get you planning on how to conduct your clinical education research and disseminate your hard work.

We know that what you are about to read will be something that you will cover over the period of months (or more!). But we trust you will read the workbook, make some plans, and then come back to individual chapters as you engage with your path in the research cycle!

Enjoy taking some time to consider your research journey! We believe you have so much to contribute.

*—Mark and Sarah*

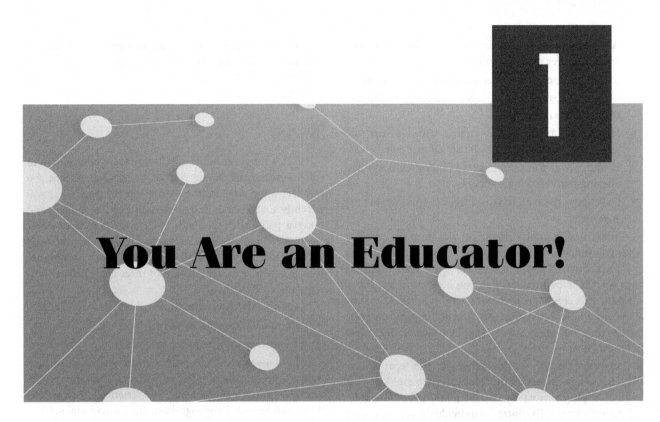

# You Are an Educator!

*Mark DeRuiter, MBA, PhD, CCC-A/SLP, F-ASHA*
*and Sarah M. Ginsberg, EdD, CCC-SLP, F-ASHA*

We came to higher education after being full-time clinicians (speech-language pathology and audiology) for multiple years. That work involved clinical activities but also nurturing the next generation of clinicians through mentorship and career guidance. Over time, both of us came to work in higher education roles that involved activities even more keenly focused on supporting the future clinicians of our discipline. Both of us have distinct memories of being given some form to complete that asked us to identify our professions. We recall waffling for a ridiculously long time: Were we speech-language pathologists/audiologists who educated student clinicians, or were we educators who taught in communication sciences and disorders? Our professional identities had first been defined by clinical roles; however, the longer we spent working with graduate student clinicians, as clinical educators and in the classroom, we felt our identities shift a bit to focus on our expanded knowledge about both clinical work and educational work. Eventually both of us came to identify primarily as educators.

This chapter is designed to get you thinking about some of the roles you play in your career and how you are connected to clinical education. We'd like to get you thinking about the variety of ways you may have served as an educator along the way—perhaps without even knowing it. We hope that you will take some time to reflect and consider other roles that we may not have included in this chapter, too. The chapter certainly isn't all-inclusive. Instead, think of it like a lens through which you might view the subsequent chapters of this workbook.

## CLINICIANS EDUCATING

You are an educator! Have you ever thought about this statement? It's what this whole book is about. For some of us, the label of educator might be greeted with enthusiasm thinking of a role in a school or higher education environment. For others, it might be more of a stretch. However, if you are working to educate the next generation of clinicians, *you are an educator.* This role can come in many forms:

DeRuiter, M., & Ginsberg, S. M. (Eds.). *Clinician's Guide to Applying,*
*Conducting, and Disseminating Clinical Education Research* (pp. 1-7).
© 2024 Taylor & Francis Group.

- Accepting a novice clinician into your clinical practice as an observer or active student clinician
- Offering a guest lecture for a university-level course
- Supporting students through mentoring in state- or national-level programs
- Having a spontaneous conversation with a learner who you meet casually or at a professional meeting
- Looking over the resume of a budding clinician and offering pointers for job success
- Describing the path to your career or specialty area to a learner

These few examples might get you thinking of other ways you influence the next generation of clinicians. This is a great time to pause and reflect upon your influence because it may be broader than you have considered it in the past. This chapter is written to get you to think broadly about your role as an educator, and subsequent chapters take a voice that infers your role *as an educator and potential researcher*.

In case you are wondering, we use the term *clinical educator* to encompass all professionals who are doing the work of helping *novice clinicians* learn how to become independent clinicians. This includes individuals who may work in a university clinic full-time with student clinicians and those who work in the community settings and only spend a part of their time with students or work with students intermittently. We use the clinical educator label because we think that "supervisor" undervalues the role that clinical educators play in the educational process. Throughout this book, you will also see us refer to *novice clinicians*. This term is intended to be interpreted broadly and take into account any individual who is not yet fully independent in their clinical practice. That might be an undergraduate or graduate student, an intern, or a resident, depending on your profession.

So think of yourself as a clinical educator, and all the other roles you might have in your day-to-day work life. Some of us are excited to consider new roles. Others are hesitant to take on anything new or different in our sphere. We might feel overloaded, overlooked, or overwhelmed. Let's think through the various roles of a clinician and the different ways you might consider your day.

# ROLES YOU MAY HOLD AND WHY THEY ARE IMPORTANT

## Employee

You are an employee of an organization (or perhaps an employee-owner). In this role, you are accountable to the people you serve and the organization as a whole. Serving as an employee is how most of us get paid, and it might be what we are most comfortable considering because it pays the bills!

## Clinician

In this role, you use the skills you were educated in to treat the variety of people you serve. This role pushes you to reflect upon what you've learned in the past, what you currently understand, and what you need to understand to serve patients/clients with issues you may have never encountered before. You do this by using evidence-based practice (EBP). As you might recall, EBP gives us a framework to consider the integration of three areas in our clinical practice. These include:

- Clinical expertise/opinion
- Internal and external evidence
- Patient/caregiver perspectives

These areas are often presented as a triangle to help us think holistically about our patients, their needs, the extant literature, and what we've experienced as clinicians (American Speech-Language-Hearing Association, n.d.).

For some of us, considering EBP immediately takes us back to graduate school and the strong push our programs instilled in us to reinforce our clinical work with evidence. It might also bring back memories of asking "PICO questions" as we considered our cases. The PICO framework is a mnemonic, which includes asking questions related to health care problems in the following way:

- Patient, problem, or population
- Intervention
- Comparison/control
- Outcome

Asking a question using this framework might help us frame our literature search and shape the way we treat a patient. We're including an example in this chapter, but you will find many other opportunities to engage with the PICO framework throughout this workbook.

## BOX 1-1: PICO CLINICAL EDUCATION EXAMPLE

**P:** Graduate students in hospital setting
**I:** Learn how to assess client bedside for presence of dysphagia
**C:** Practice with simulation vs. practice with patients
**O:** Graduate student independence in completing clinical screening

For some of us, thinking about the EBP framework and PICO questions might be something we found onerous and overly specific. Others may have found the process energizing and a way to feed their curiosity. This entire workbook is to help you consider the helpful "middle" of EBP and subsequent PICO questions, and to stretch your thinking beyond the patient care triangle and consider our evidence in how we educate students.

## Researcher

This one might feel like a bit of a leap for clinicians. However, it fits well with your clinician role. When faced with a novel clinical scenario, instead of stating you cannot serve a potential client/patient because they exhibit something that is new to you, you start exploring. You use the tools that you have available to you to find out how to best serve the person. You research by using books, articles, internet searches, and conversations with other colleagues who may point you to resources you hadn't considered before. The point is: You are a clinician-researcher in your exploration—and you are likely using the tools of EBP and PICO questions! But the researcher element doesn't stop there. You are also a researcher when you engage with your patients/clients. You form hypotheses and you test those hypotheses. You review the data you've collected and determine when you need to change course. You'll gather further information necessary to change your plan of action using the aforementioned strategies. The important element here is that, as a clinician-researcher, you don't give up. Instead, you find ways to assist those you serve by asking and answering questions.

## Person With Limits on Time and Energy

We'd be remiss if we didn't mention this important foundational element of the many roles in which you serve. All of us hold a variety of roles and the work of our days does not end when we leave the office, school, or clinic. Instead, we move on to other responsibilities in our personal spheres. This can make the time required to learn or do something new seem daunting. Our best hope for you is that you will find ways to create the time and energy needed to engage with this workbook and your activities with the next generation of clinicians.

# How the Roles Might Fit Together

If you think about the variety of ways you may have educated others and then nest them with your various professional and personal roles, you can begin to consider how these elements might come together. For those of us who serve in a role of *clinical educator*, you will likely be able to conceptually merge clinician, employee, and accepting a student into your clinical practice as a logical connection. However, how does research impact that relationship? It certainly has an impact when you consider EBP and working through best options for the person you will serve alongside your student clinician. But what do we know about how we educate our students who are the next generation of clinicians? Have you stopped to consider what research might be available to you and where you might access that work? These questions get us thinking on a different level. We're going to start off by telling you right now: There is a dearth of research available regarding clinical education in the discipline of communication sciences and disorders. Does that mean there is none? Of course not, but there is much more we need to learn and many creative questions we can ask. The inquisitive lens that we use for working with clients/patients shifts to something that we might be less familiar with when we think about working with a student, mainly because we might not have been pushed to think this way before.

---

## Box 1-2:
### Looking Outside Your Discipline

The reality of the situation is that there might be many answers relative to research in student education in some disciplines (e.g., nursing, physician, education) and a paucity of information in other disciplines (e.g., audiology and speech-language pathology). As you ponder this, you might consider the ways health care education might look differently across disciplines based on the type of service as well (i.e., some areas will be habilitative or rehabilitative whereas others might offer one-time treatments to deal with patient needs). Therefore, information from one discipline might not always "fit" another, and this could be true across patient-centered EBP, as well as student-centered evidence-based education (EBE) practice (Ginsberg et al., 2012).

---

# Evidence-Based Education–Clinical Education Model

DeRuiter and Ginsberg (2020) provided a model that might help you think about EBP, EBE, and other factors relative to your role as a clinical educator and put it all together. Let's dissect each portion of the evidence-based education-clinical education (EBE-CE) model next (Figure 1-1). On the left side of the model, we have the figure that represents our fundamental clinical work and addresses our EBP

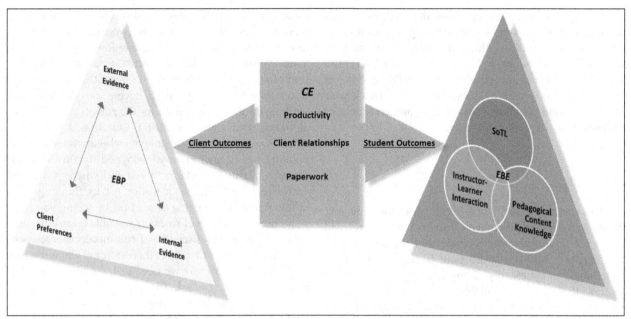

**Figure 1-1.** The EBE-CE model. (Reproduced with permission from DeRuiter, M., & Ginsberg, S. M. [2020]. Conscious clinical education: The evidence-based education-clinical education model. *Seminars in Speech-Language Pathology, Special Topics Issue*. https://doi.org/10.1055 /s-0040-1713779)

(American Speech-Language-Hearing Association, n.d.). These aspects of our roles are the ones we are most familiar with in our daily clinical work. Most of us focus our professional development (see the left-hand side of Figure 1-1 and think about your continuing education relative to your day-to-day practice) in this domain on approaches to assessment or treatment of a disorder where the assessment/treatment approach is new or the disorder is one we have less experience with.

Moving to the right side of the model, we have the work that has often been associated with classroom learning but is really about teaching and learning in general. This side of the model represents the EBE aspect of our work and begins to combine our clinical work into the clinical education realm (Ginsberg et al., 2012). On this side, our knowledge and skills relate to the content that we are teaching novice clinicians, the process of teaching and learning, and our understanding of instructor-learner interactions.

The three key elements of the EBE model might be new to you, but they will help you to become a better clinical educator as you learn more about them (DeRuiter & Ginsberg, 2020; Ginsberg & DeRuiter, 2020; Ginsberg et al., 2012).

1. Scholarship of teaching and learning (SoTL): SoTL refers to a body of research that informs best practices in higher education. It can be described as systematic, high-quality research that informs us of the best practices for education. SoTL research examines learner characteristics, teaching approaches, and the context of teaching and learning. By conducting and reading this type of research, we learn about the best ways in which to prepare future clinicians.

2. Pedagogical content knowledge: Pedagogical content knowledge refers to the combined insights that an instructor has regarding the clinical knowledge they are trying to impart and how best to explain it to the learner (Shulman, 1998).

3. Instructor-learner interaction: Information in this area focuses on the knowledge that each participant in the process has about the other. This might include, for example, what the instructor knows about the student (e.g., they are a graduate student who was just admitted to their clinical preparation program vs. they are a graduate student who is about to complete their clinical preparation program and enter the field) and what the learner understands about the instructor (e.g., they are open to new ideas; the instructor is approachable).

The right side of this model might be new to you—and that is just fine. It is a big part of a workbook like this one, and you'll find ways that each chapter of this workbook fits with this side of the model, whether you are consuming, producing, or simply wondering about research in the clinical education space. For now, we encourage you to pause a moment and reflect on it, making a commitment to refer back to it as you move along.

Finally, consider the elements in the middle of Figure 1-1. We've included a few examples there, but there could be many more. We like to think of these as "hidden factors" because they are not always at the surface or predictable. There are many different things that influence your practice with a patient *and* a student clinician. This will be highly dynamic and something that changes dependent upon the individual situation. For instance, you may have a relationship with your given patient and having a student in your clinical space might impact that relationship. This could cause you, your patient, and the student some stress as roles are realigned in the clinical environment. Alternatively, you might have particular productivity demands in your clinical environment that shape how you work and how you interact with a student clinician. There are a whole variety of hidden factors, and not all of them need to be negative. The point here is to get you thinking that as an educator, there is much you will need to consider along the way, and it might be variable across patients and learners.

## Navigating Patient Preferences: A Critical Hidden Factor

Faculty who work in higher education are programmed to focus on the needs of their students. However, in clinical environments, we know that the sphere widens. Navigating patient preferences in the clinical sphere is paramount. This supersedes student preference and it's important to novice clinicians that it's entirely clear you will do what you can to support their learning, within the confines of keeping patients safe and supporting efficient patient appointments.

We discussed this preference in our work in 2020 (DeRuiter & Ginsberg) and touched on it before, and it brings us back to some "hidden factors" that can be implied in Figure 1-1. There is a significant amount of navigation in this realm. One area is what was previously mentioned, the question of whether a patient is willing to work with a student clinician. This should be an informed decision for the patient/family with a thorough understanding of your role as a clinician in managing the care. A layer deeper for some clinicians can be "letting go" of their own patients and having a triangulated space with the student clinician who likely is with you for a short period of time. For some clinicians, this is more challenging than others.

Another factor can be navigating the EBP itself. You'll be working with a student who is likely highly focused on evidence-based treatments as they have learned about them in the classroom. However, what might be more complex is when your patient rejects evidence-based approaches/treatments for another option. This will put you in conversation with both your patient and your student clinician. The student will be a partner who may need to see your example for how you navigate these complex conversations and maintain relationships with the patient. It is important to have these conversations so that students understand "best" recommendations, as well as working within the confines of patient preferences. Through observing a difficult conversation, your student clinician might possibly walk away with enduring knowledge that you might take for granted.

## SUMMING IT UP

Figure 1-1 helps you put together a variety of ways that you might work, think, and develop yourself as a clinical educator. We will talk much more about this as we move through this workbook. For now, pause and reflect on the big picture of student education and make a list of what feels comfortable and uncomfortable to you in the context of student education. Next, list out what you are most curious about learning relative to being a clinical educator. You'll want to come back to these lists after you finish with this manual, and consider where you have grown and where more opportunities still exist for you!

## REFERENCES

American Speech-Language-Hearing Association. (n.d.). *Evidence-based practice (EBP)*. Author. Retrieved July 25, 2022, from https://www.asha.org/research/ebp/

DeRuiter, M., & Ginsberg, S. M. (2020). Conscious clinical education: The evidence-based education-clinical education model. *Seminars in Speech and Language, 41*(4), 279-288. https://doi.org/10.1055/s-0040-1713779

Ginsberg, S. M., & DeRuiter, M. (2020). Research and the clinical education and supervision process. In E. S. McCrae & J. A. Brasseur (Eds.), *The clinical education and supervisory process in speech-language pathology and audiology* (pp. 411-426). SLACK Incorporated.

Ginsberg, S. M., Friberg, J. C., & Visconti, C. (2012). *Scholarship of teaching and learning in speech-language pathology and audiology: Evidence-based education*. Plural Publishing, Inc.

Shulman, L. S. (1998). Introduction. In P. Hutchings (Ed.), *The course portfolio: How faculty can examine their teaching to advance practice and improve student learning* (pp. 5-12). Stylus.

*Worksheet Note: After each chapter you will find a worksheet. The worksheets are connected to the chapter's content, and they are also designed to move your thinking about your research forward.*

# Worksheet 1-1:
# You Are an Educator

What are some of the ways in which you support and educate the next generation of clinicians?

Are there ways in which you would like to work with novice clinicians in the future?

## Professional Roles

What roles do you play in your setting and how do these roles require you to also be an educator?

| Role | Education Process |
|---|---|
| Employee | |
| Clinician | |
| Researcher | |
| Clinical educator | |
| Other | |

*(continued)*

# Worksheet 1-1:
# You Are an Educator (continued)

**EBE-CE Model**

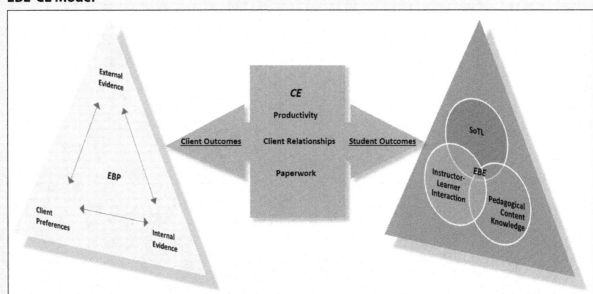

What aspects of your work depicted in this model raise questions for you?
[Tip: List all questions that come to mind—you will sort later.]

Where do you see important intersections that feel like areas you might want to research?

# 2

# Teaching and Learning in Clinical Education

*Sarah M. Ginsberg, EdD, CCC-SLP, F-ASHA*
*and Mark DeRuiter, MBA, PhD, CCC-A/SLP, F-ASHA*

This chapter is designed to get you thinking about taxonomies of learning, design for teaching and learning, and putting these elements together in the context of a real-world environment. There is much to consider here, and it is impossible to have this be all-inclusive. Instead, the goal is to have you thinking broadly about what we know about teaching and learning and how you might apply it in the context of student learning. If you have set this workbook down for a bit (and you may have!), look back at Chapter 1. In that chapter, we referred to an evidence-based education model of clinical education. Much of the content in this chapter will focus on information related to this part of the model. On the right side of the model, we referred to three different areas. These were:

1. Scholarship of teaching and learning: Scholarship of teaching and learning refers to a body of research that informs best practices in higher education. It can be described as systematic, high-quality research that informs us of the best practices for education.

2. Pedagogical content knowledge: Pedagogical content knowledge refers to the combined insights that an instructor has regarding the clinical knowledge they are trying to impart and how best to explain it to the learner (Shulman, 1998).

3. Instructor-learner interaction: Information in this area focuses on the knowledge that each participant in the process has about the other.

If these aren't "small reminders" for you, you might want to travel back to Chapter 1 and refresh your knowledge. Otherwise, you are ready to move forward and take your thinking up a level (or many levels!) to consider frameworks that influence how we might consider learning within clinical education about student education. You might wonder, "But, why?" We feel strongly that considering things like taxonomies of learning, design for teaching and learning, and putting these elements together in the context of a real-world environment will help you begin thinking about your own research questions. Over time, you'll find other resources and frameworks, and we encourage you to do so. However, let's get you started with some core elements from which you will grow.

DeRuiter, M., & Ginsberg, S. M. (Eds.). *Clinician's Guide to Applying, Conducting, and Disseminating Clinical Education Research* (pp. 9-19).

# FOUNDATIONAL KNOWLEDGE: TAXONOMIES OF LEARNING

## Bloom's Taxonomy

Probably one of the most familiar learning taxonomies is Bloom's taxonomy. This taxonomy is often presented as a pyramid and has its roots back into the 1950s (Bloom, 1956). The base of the pyramid deals with remembering facts and moves through multiple other layers to peak at evaluation. The layers (from the bottom up) include:

- Knowledge
- Comprehension
- Application
- Analysis
- Synthesis
- Evaluation

The entire hierarchy can be divided into categories of higher- and lower-order thinking. An example of lower-order thinking might be a student memorizing a procedure in your clinical environment (the "knowledge" element of the pyramid). However, as a student engages with that procedure, they may come to you with questions demonstrating deep consideration of what they are learning. For instance, the student may *analyze* when to use the procedure, *synthesize its application* appropriately, and even *evaluate* the use of the procedure. This could be evident during your conversations.

Considering that Bloom's taxonomy has many elements that make sense to many of us, we want to keep it in our repertoire of taxonomies because it has been heavily used in education at all grade levels. The work of Bloom has been modified over time, too. In the 1990s to early 2000s, Anderson (2005) and colleagues modified the taxonomy to change the names of the layers to verb forms and rearrange the order a bit to acknowledge more active thinking and learning during the educational process. Particularly, this work acknowledged an affective domain to address how a learner might feel, value, appreciate, and be motivated by what they are learning. This affective element was based on previous work of Krathwohl and colleagues (1973). It is important to keep in mind because a wide range of studies have demonstrated that how learners feel about the learning experience can significantly influence their learning and their attitudes toward what they learned.

This type of change reflects that there may be other ways to consider learning for our students and their role in the process. Therefore, let's move forward with other taxonomies so you understand other options that might not always be considered in health care disciplines.

## Miller's Pyramid of Assessment

We'll review Miller's Pyramid of Assessment (Miller, 1990) next because it has some elements that fit naturally with Bloom's work, as well as some real-world implications. Miller posited that medical education should focus not just on knowledge but also testing that knowledge in real-world environments. Miller's pyramid has four different hierarchical processes to consider clinical competence. At the bottom (lowest) level of the pyramid is "knowledge." Knowledge is easily assessed with things like written examinations and can be demonstrated with activities like fill-in-the-blank answers or multiple-choice questions. Next on the hierarchy is "application of knowledge." Application can be demonstrated by completing essay questions, discussing a clinical problem-solving exercise with a mentoring clinician, or extended case-based multiple-choice questions. The third tier represents "clinical competency." For some fields, this may be assessed using methods that are new to some of us. Here, students might engage with simulations, standardized patients, or other clinical examinations. The final tier, "clinical performance," is observing performance of a student clinician within the clinical environment.

Sim and colleagues (2015) have encouraged us to think about the lower two tiers of the hierarchy as cognitive and the upper tiers as behavioral. As you consider your own clinical training, you might see that you engaged in a "behaviorist" model such as this one. Although your performance in coursework mattered (cognitive), if you were not able to perform in clinic (behavioral), you would likely not pass through your program. The same is true for

---

# BOX 2-1: BLOOM'S TAXONOMY APPLIED

- **Knowledge:** A student learns about the procedure, remembering it in a linear order of events.

- **Comprehension:** The student watches the procedure completed and starts to comprehend the need for the steps. They can explain why each step is taken.

- **Application:** The student begins to use the information and can demonstrate conducting it in a real-world environment.

- **Analysis:** The student distinguishes the importance of various aspects of the procedure and may experiment with different ways to complete it most effectively.

- **Synthesis:** The student begins determining the best way to conduct the procedure, particularly for different patients, to achieve the best outcome. They can justify why changes in steps or modifications are most appropriate for a given patient.

- **Evaluation:** The student develops their own approach to the procedure and can explain how and why it works to others.

## BOX 2-2:
## MILLER'S PYRAMID OF ASSESSMENT APPLIED

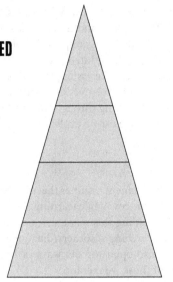

- **Clinical performance:** Student conducts the procedure with a real patient.

- **Clinical competency:** Student executes the procedure in a simulation-based laboratory setting.

- **Application of knowledge:** Student describes how steps in procedure might be completed for a fictional case.

- **Knowledge:** Student lists steps in a procedure on a written test.

Data source: Miller, G. E. (1990). The assessment of clinical skills/competence/performance. *Academic Medicine: Journal of the Association of American Medical Colleges, 65*(9 Suppl), S63-S67.

students who exhibited poor performance in class (cognitive) but had a natural ability engaging patients in a clinical setting (behavior). Although building rapport and working well with patients is an asset, it is not the only element that makes a clinician.

Miller's work (1990) is another useful way for us to think about how students learn and how they might be assessed in classroom and clinical settings, and it might take us slightly deeper than what we can consider with Bloom's taxonomy. With Miller's work, we begin to consider the application of knowledge and how it could be assessed in the clinical environment.

## *Fink's Significant Learning Outcomes*

Shift your thinking now from something more linear (i.e., hierarchies, cognitive complexity, behavioral domains) to thinking about your novice clinician out in the world. We know that when our students engage with new information out in a real environment, they may piece things together in a nonlinear way. Considering this, we can think about novice clinicians who have different clinical education experiences, yet all have a final ending point or competency. How could this be done given a variety of ways the student might learn material, the differences across clinical populations, and variety in clinical learning environments? This is where Fink's taxonomy might be useful.

Fink (2003) addressed creating significant learning in a way that looks at overlapping yet contributing elements that can be organized in six different ways. These are:

### Foundational Knowledge

Here you can think of remembering and understanding foundational knowledge for clinical practice.

### Application

This element moves into thinking about how to apply foundational knowledge into different contexts. What is important here is that a learner can be challenged to think about the application of foundational knowledge in new and different ways.

### Integration

At this point the learner starts "putting it together." Some of us can see this start to happen with our students in their practice and conversations. They start to talk with us about what they have learned elsewhere and how the pieces fit across the people they serve and various environments.

### Human Dimension

With this element, learners are considering how the information they are learning applies to them and the people they serve. This can be very powerful. Learners also think about themselves and how their success (or failure) could impact their self-image or self-ideal. This element is an excellent example of one that is continually operating for the learning, regardless of their experience level.

## Caring

The element of caring assumes that the learner cares about the content and understands why they should care. We might make assumptions that our learners come to study their field of interest because they care. However, we should never make assumptions. Some may feel nudged to go to school by relatives or significant others. Other learners could be going through the motions. (As a mentor, you can help make caring explicit for a novice clinician).

## Learning How to Learn

This element assumes that our students will refine their learning process while learning. As a clinician, you're doing this by reading this manual, learning about new technologies, researching disorders/diagnoses, and so on. However, you're also open to new ways of learning. We expect the same of those we mentor.

---

### Box 2-3: Fink's Creating Significant Learning Applied

- **Foundational knowledge:** The student is able to understand and explain the steps for the procedure.
- **Application:** The student is able to analyze the clinical scenario described in a case and differentiate how they might complete the procedure in the given situation.
- **Integration:** The student makes connections between patients seen in a different setting and synthesizes their new knowledge of how to complete the procedure with that type of patient.
- **Human dimension:** The student learns how to effectively explain the procedure to the patient prior to doing it such that they can reduce the patient's anxiety and express empathy for how the patient is feeling about the impending procedure.
- **Caring:** The student feels excitement about becoming a skilled professional capable of completing the procedure.
- **Learning how to learn:** The student reflects on their performance conducting the procedure and explores mechanisms for improving their skills.

---

Fink's continuum of learning creates an exciting way to consider learning holistically. It's arguably less linear and can ignite conversations with those around us about how we do what we do when we learn and mentor others. It also might get us thinking about how we structure learning differently. We would argue that this could mean we structure experiences for our students less "linearly" based on what we want them to know and how they might need to perform in the future.

What is important to consider here is that unlike the models previously described, these elements must work together to facilitate the most significant learning possible. It is also important to note that this taxonomy incorporates the affective and reflective aspects of learning right into the experiences. As a psychologist-colleague recently said to me, "It is important to know yourself." Fink's model builds on this concept and focuses appreciable attention on aspects of the learning that reside within the learner, including their own values and their insights into their own learning process. Fink advocated that it is important to incorporate these principles into planning the learning experiences in order for them to be effective.

Considering frameworks like these will help you as you engage with novice clinicians and their learning needs. They might also help you consider your own research questions along the way. That leads us to thinking about designing instructional experiences, which is covered next.

# Designing for Teaching and Learning

Now let's discuss designing for teaching and learning. Regardless of which taxonomy of learning you might find most comfortable, carefully designing a learning experience can be considered critical to the success of learning. When you engage with a novice clinician in your environment, do you take the time to think about designing the experience for them? Your initial response might be "No," or "Not particularly" and you would not be alone. However, think about the questions you might ask of the novice clinician and their program before you agree to the experience:

- What level is the student?
- What courses have they had?
- What other experiences does the student bring to the table?
- What are the student's career objectives?

We have often thought of these types of questions as setting expectations. However, we argue that they are decidedly something more. You are already engaging in a process (whether you have thought about it or not!) of designing a learning experience. With answers to the aforementioned questions (and many others) you may be informally putting together an experience in your mind. The answers help you shape that design and provide input into how you might assess the student. For some clinicians, this might feel very natural. For others, it might take some deep thinking and time. This could be particularly true if an answer to a question is unexpected.

Wiggins and McTighe (2005) encourage us to think of ourselves as *designers as well as teachers*. They have linked discussions of their design process to the work of Stephen Covey (1989), with a quote many of us are familiar with:

> To begin with the end in mind means to start with a clear understanding of your destination. It means to know where you're going so that you better understand where you are now so that the steps you take are always in the right direction.
>
> —Stephen Covey, *The Seven Habits of Highly Effective People*

Wiggins and McTighe encourage us to consider a three-step design process that begins with identifying your desired results *first*. Engaging this way gets us to consider something called "backward design" where we begin with the end in mind and work backward to shape the student experience based upon desired results and assessment tools. The process is often broken into three steps, which we have demonstrated graphically in Figure 2-1 (with a focus on a clinical environment).

We describe each of these three elements further in the following, because they are critical to the process.

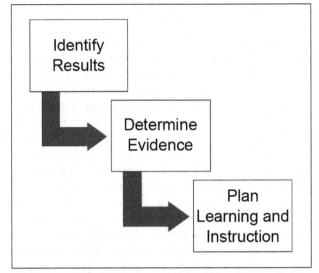

**Figure 2-1.** Backward design process. (Adapted from Wiggins, G., & McTighe, J. [2005]. *Understanding by design* [2nd ed.]. Association for Supervision and Curriculum Development.)

## Stage 1: Identify Results

What do you expect the student you are working with to be able to do by the end of the experience? This question could be wrapped up a few different ways. For instance, a university program that a student attends might be considering this question on a broad curricular level, considering how a student will be "licensure-ready" by the end of the experience. However, the experience you might be planning in a clinical setting could be different, depending upon where the student is at in their learning and how close they are to finishing their entire degree experience. For most clinical educators, you'll need to consider both the "near and far" ends of the results continuum. Additionally, most of us will agree that considering previous student experience as they enter into your clinical environment will have a bearing on what results you expect.

You can tell that Stage 1 is critical because here you are making many different decisions involving what you want your learner to know by the time you have completed your learning opportunity with them. Wiggins and McTighe have a conceptual framework for this as well. It involves three nested spheres with "enduring knowledge" in the middle and "important to know and do" and "worth being familiar with" as rings that move from the center. *Enduring knowledge* are those elements that are critical in your environment. For a clinician, this might involve understanding the fundamentals of why we engage in evaluation and treatment for the population served. Concepts of reliability and validity may also be elements at this level, as well as broad

concepts of evidence-based practice. If you're interested in Wiggins and McTighe's conceptual framework, you can learn more about it from Bowen (2017) and Sample (2011).

## Levels of Knowledge

Things that are *important to know and do* can feel close to home for clinicians. Here you can think about mastery of skill with assessment and criterion-referenced instruments. We would expect a student to be able to use and explain how these areas might overlap and yet each yield unique contributions to the clinical "picture" for the patient. Knowing and doing within treatment could also be demonstrating an understanding of cueing hierarchies and strategies and what they mean in the context of the patients served and their needs. We should also consider a learner taking content and using it appropriately in this arena.

Finally, there are things *worth being familiar with* for a learner. This could be content where we believe a learner should be conversant about a topic but maybe not develop their skills to a finely honed point. For instance, a new clinician working in a health care setting should have some fundamental understanding of health care economics and how the payment system works. However, this is a very complex area that would require a great deal of study from a learner in order for them to become an expert in the area.

You can see that Stage 1 is very broad and requires deep thought as you work with your first student clinician or two. This can be why some clinicians develop a real comfort level with working with students from the same academic program who are at the same level in their educational experience. Similar scenarios create a comfort level because you have a framework for your planning and can adjust accordingly, dependent upon the learner.

## Stage 2: Determine Evidence

After you have pulled together results, how will you know when your student has met your goal and achieved your desired result? For some clinicians, this can be addressed with a broad brushstroke: *When the student is able to take on my cases with consultation only.* However, a goal like that one would likely only fit for students who are nearly finished in their formal academic process. What about other learners? You might have set particular goals for scoring assessments, writing chart notes and reports, or navigating treatment for patients with specific diagnoses. You'll also consult documentation from a university or national organization to determine what assessment tools might be available for you in meeting your goals at a given point in time (more on this in a bit).

The previously mentioned results could be formalized and tracked using an electronic system or pen and paper. However, you could even set goals around student performance in discussing their cases and develop a gestalt assessment over time as well. Here you could assess their planning and reflective abilities to see what they know (e.g., you could ask reflective questions after a session, such as, "What would you have done if *x* had happened? Why?") Keep in mind, you want to be clear in what the goal is so that your learner has a complete understanding of the expectations. Most importantly, your acceptable evidence needs to be directly linked to your desired result. Without this link, your evidence may be considered arbitrary.

If you are new to the world of mentoring novice clinicians, you might want to start with tools the university has given you. You'll often find there is an electronic system or other form you will use to rate student performance. You could begin your backward-planning from here by determining what form your environment is covered in the assessment and then adding additional elements of your own—as specific learning goals for the student clinician. Just remember, you will want to give your student a voice in this process, too. There may be particular elements of practice they find more or less challenging. These elements might shape your acceptable evidence.

## Stage 3: Plan Learning and Instruction

The last step is to pull everything together. Here you review your enduring knowledge, important to know and understand, and worth being familiar with the elements, and you start mapping them to your assessment types and your environment. This is where the backward design is really taking place because you are also considering what opportunities exist in your clinical environment for teaching and learning and how you will expand upon them.

This might appear daunting initially. If it feels that way, it likely means that you are doing it right! It is very likely that not every element will occur across each of your patients or even your work week for that matter. You might also find that some opportunities are abundant, and others are lean. If some opportunities are fewer within a given time period, you might think about other ways for the student to gain knowledge and skill (and for you to assess that knowledge and skill). This could be through working alongside another clinician who has more opportunities, simulating experiences, engaging in deep conversations about specific content areas, or more. Another thing to consider here is what your student believes they need from the experience with you. Interviewing the student and determining what they see as the future of the experience can be enlightening and help you shape your objectives and assessments.

Think for a moment about those previous statements. What is your focus? It might feel broad and moving beyond making certain that you are ready to mind the process and check the boxes. Why? The answer is because you are thinking about this new clinician and everything they need to know and what it will take for them to start out in their career. This is definitely much more than a discrete set of skills and might feel like an area that is difficult for you to even put into words. You have moved into broad goals, and you've gained student input to determine your steps in the process and you're already thinking about the student's future. What you have done here is move from instruction alone to thinking about student learning.

### Box 2-4: Simplified Backward Design Example With a Novice Clinician

- **Stage 1—Identify Results:** Given student experience level, they will be able to handle "non-complex" patients on the clinician's workload by the end of the semester with minimal assistance.

- **Stage 2—Determine Evidence:** This will be evidenced by fading prompts from the clinical educator in the room. By the end of the semester, the clinical educator will intervene no more than one time during each treatment session with non-complex patients.

- **Stage 3—Plan Learning and Instruction:** The clinical educator will:

  ○ Confirm goals with the university program

  ○ Interview the student to establish shared learning goals

  ○ Begin with a student observation period of 1 week

  ○ Release non-complex patients to the students gradually, over weeks 2 through 4

  ○ Fade prompts during weeks 5 through 12, while collecting data on the nature and type of prompts

  ○ Adjust as necessary

# EMPOWERING YOUR STUDENTS: BARR AND TAGG

We use "instruction" and "training" infrequently. Instead, you might notice words like "learning," "knowledge," and "education" more often. This is because we have a bias toward thinking about learner-centric activities where students learn and are actively engaged in the process. This concept isn't new and much of it is a reflection of the work of Barr and Tagg (1995).

Reflect on your own learning for a moment. How much of it was spent in a traditional form of instruction? You can think of traditional instruction as a time where you had closely defined meeting times (usually whole hours) where faculty stood at the front of the room and delivered lectures. For many of us, this was a traditional form of education where we may have felt very comfortable. Barr and Tagg worked to challenge this notion. Think of how your learning could have been different if, rather than instructing you, faculty empowered you to learn and set the stage for that to happen? This might mean significantly less lecture content and more time for you to interact with what you are learning and forging a path to better understand what you need to know, without a "sage on the stage" to tell you where you are going.

This shift from instruction/lecture to learning is exactly what Barr and Tagg discussed in their work. If you think about it, it could possibly be close to clinical learning. As a clinician, you likely spend much less time "lecturing" to a student clinician. Instead, you spend time planning and nurturing them to dive into the ocean of learning where you might serve more as a coach than an instructor per se. You know that you cannot anticipate every challenge your student will face as they engage with a patient population. Instead, you prepare them as best you can and then support them in finding and developing resources— whether those resources are external or internal to themselves.

Barr and Tagg (1995) view instruction through a lens where the educator is the center of the atom. In the preferred learning paradigm, knowledge is at the center of the atom with both educators and learners approaching and interacting with that knowledge. It is definitely a different approach than many of us may have experienced in the classroom. Higher education continues to make this shift making classrooms more interactive and collaborative. This requires more effort on the part of the learner to engage and examine what they know and have yet to learn. As you interact with student clinicians you might find some who will tell you they are more comfortable learning in the classroom and others learning in the clinic (and some who are comfortable in both!). This is likely because these two environments are still very distinct for them in their educational approaches. However, know that as a clinical educator you are at the cutting edge of operating in how students engage and learn—this is by putting information into practice and testing what they know and do not know. Some may be more comfortable collaborating and learning than others.

# PUTTING IT ALL TOGETHER

So far we have talked about your role as an educator, taxonomies of learning, designing teaching and learning, and how our lens on learning might be shifting over time. With each area of discussion, we hope we have encouraged you to think on an increasingly higher level about education, how we learn, and how the paradigm might be shifting overall in the context of education. Now, let's consider some ways this information gets put into practice.

## Student Learning Objectives: Going Beyond the Objectives

Although we might be nudged to think of categories of learning (e.g., disorder areas, instrumental vs. behavioral assessments), we are going to encourage you to think even more broadly as you engage with students. Our hope is that this chapter has inspired you to consider broad, enduring knowledge that your learner needs to understand in the clinical environment where you work. Although a university or national assessment form might not include a category like this, it is worthwhile to step back and determine what it will take for your student to move from learner to licensed professional who is a lifelong learner. How can you instill both curiosity and critical evaluation of resources for your student clinician? It will likely be by modeling these behaviors very deliberately as a first step. Then, you will want to consider the different experiences that might be required for you to engage the learner to develop their curiosity and self-advocacy. And, surprisingly for some, you don't necessarily always have to be in the same room with the learner to get this to happen. Instead, you can inspire them to take on planned challenges in your environment where they can continue to safely grow and learn.

Part of this growth will come from you encouraging the learner to take part in their own learning process. Give them time to observe your environment so they can see what you do and how you operate. Before observation begins, let them know that you are seeking structured thoughts on what they would like to learn that goes beyond what they have discovered in the classroom and other clinical experiences. This will help you negotiate goals with the student clinician and set appropriate expectations. Does this mean you won't use forms assigned to you from the university? No, we're not suggesting that. But we are encouraging you to move the learner to take active ownership of what they are learning when they are engaged with you. This will likely be a significant shift from their classroom experience. For some, it might feel uncomfortable. That is why you need to give the student time to reflect and understand that their goals will be greeted with enthusiasm.

---

## BOX 2-5:
### STUDENT CLINICAL LEARNING OBJECTIVES

Student learning objectives can come in a whole variety of forms. We often talk about how clinical learning objectives could warrant a whole textbook unto themselves! But if learning objectives are new to you, here are some examples to get you thinking:

- Student will independently choose, administer, and score norm-referenced assessments for patients with [insert category] disorder.

- Student will make appropriate hearing aid recommendations for patients with mild-to-moderate sensorineural hearing loss with minimal support after 6 weeks of clinic exposure.

- Student will independently present assessment findings in an individualized education program meeting in weeks 14 to 15 of the semester.

- Student will independently collect patient histories for [insert category] disorder after 7 weeks of clinic exposure.

You might start picking these objectives apart with thoughts like, "But, these could be clearer or more granular." If this is where your mind is going, bravo! We can't say these are "best" objectives without knowing the learner, their experience, your environment, and what is most important for the given situation. However, these can get you started as you get thinking about objectives and "big picture learning." What is most important is that you give consideration to what you want the novice clinician to be able to do at the end of their "lesson" or time with you.

---

You might also consider asking your student clinician about the approach they find most effective for their learning. For instance, some students might ask that you slowly release the reins of your patient load onto them whereas others might ask to dive into learning as quickly as possible. A short list of what you want to gather from your novice clinician here might look like this:

- How would you rate your knowledge of the clinical topic? (This might be an ongoing question as you engage with different types of clinical scenarios.)
- What is your preferred mode for feedback?
- How frequently do you require feedback?
- What response will you have if I step in as the lead clinician and take over the case during the assessment or treatment session?
- How much support do you believe you need to get started? (This may be an ongoing question as a student clinician engages with many different areas of your practice.)
- How will you signal to me that you need assistance?
- What signal would you prefer from me that I am about to step in during the session?
- What actions on my part might cause you additional stress in a clinical encounter?
- What are three ways I might support you most during the average clinical encounter?

There could be a long list of other questions, but these will get you moving forward to learning about style and preference from your learner.

Another thing we are hoping happens here is that it gets you thinking about questions. We'll have more on this workbook about questions and research. But, these frameworks, elements of design, and crafting of learning objectives are ripe with many different areas for research questions. Give yourself to wonder and think a bit about that!

## WHERE DO WE GO FROM HERE?

This chapter has given you many things to consider. You have been guided through different taxonomies of learning, design for teaching and learning, as well as ways to put this together in the context of student outcomes and navigating your complex environment. What's next?

## *Reflection*

We encourage you to step back and reflect on what you have read. If you are new to clinical education, what does this information mean to you? Has it shifted where you begin working with a novice clinician? If you are a seasoned clinical educator, how has the information presented thus far changed or challenged your thinking about the educational process? Take some time to answer these questions without interruption.

After you have reflected on the previous questions, take yourself back to thinking about research. A common link to research for clinicians is through evidence-based practice. We trust that it shapes your evaluation and treatment every single day that you find yourself in the clinical environment. One thing you will likely understand is that not all questions are answered in the literature. So, you keep searching. You might have to find the answer by doing the research yourself.

Now, step out of that space and think about clinical education. Have you taken time to consider clinical education and what research exists there? For many clinicians, the answer is, "No." That is not a fault. Instead, it can stem from a variety of reasons:

- You educate others in the same way you were educated. As a clinical educator, you may have taken the "best" of your personal experiences and worked to replicate them for a student clinician in your environment today. But do you know if these traditions work?

- You've had and have many different roles. As a student, you were focused on becoming the best clinician you could be. At work, you are carrying out that similar vision with an additional step: providing the best clinical service you can deliver. The different roles you have held/hold may not have created the time you need to research clinical education.

- Frankly, there isn't necessarily a large volume of evidence out there for clinical education, particularly for some disciplines. It's possible you have run into challenges researching what you need to know because of a paucity of data.

These reasons are what this text is about. It is to get you thinking about what *you* can contribute to the knowledge base and how you might go about doing that. The subsequent chapters are designed to get you thinking about your role as a researcher beyond clinical diagnoses alone. You will widen your perspective with practical tools to consider how you might contribute to the knowledge base of clinical education as a researcher yourself. It will be an exciting journey, and we're pleased you are joining us. The next chapters are written by experts in their fields with practical thoughts and inspiring examples. We are thrilled you've picked up this manual to take your next steps toward research in clinical education!

# REFERENCES

Anderson, L. W. (2005). Objectives, evaluation, and the improvement of education. *Studies in Educational Evaluation, 31*(2-3), 102-113. https://doi.org/10.1016/j.stueduc.2005.05.004

Barr, R. B., & Tagg, J. (1995). From teaching to learning—A new paradigm for undergraduate education. *Change, 27,* 18-25.

Bloom, B. S. (1956). *Taxonomy of educational objectives, handbook 1: Cognitive domain.* McKay.

Bowen, R. S. (2017). *Understanding by design.* Vanderbilt University Center for Teaching. https://cft.vanderbilt.edu/understanding-by-design/

Covey, S. (1989). *The seven habits of highly effective people.* Simon & Schuster.

Fink, L. D. (2003). *Creating significant learning experiences: An integrated approach to designing college courses.* Jossey-Bass.

Krathwohl, D. R., Bloom, B. S., & Masia, B. B. (1973). Taxonomy of educational objectives. *Handbook 2: Affective Domain.* Longman Group Limited.

Miller, G. E. (1990). The assessment of clinical skills/competence/performance. *Academic Medicine: Journal of the Association of American Medical Colleges, 65*(9 Suppl), S63-S67.

Sample, M. (2011). Teaching for enduring understanding. *The Chronicle of Higher Education.* https://www.chronicle.com/blogs/profhacker/teaching-for-enduring-understanding

Shulman, L. S. (1998). Introduction. In P. Hutchings (Ed.), *The course portfolio: How faculty can examine their reaching to advance practice and improve student learning* (pp. 5-12). Stylus.

Sim, J. H., Aziz, Y. F. A., Mansor, A., Vijayananthan, A., Foong, C. C., & Vadivel, J. (2015). Students' performance in the different clinical skills assessed in OSCE: What does it reveal? *Medical Education Online, 20.*

Wiggins, G., & McTighe, J. (2005). *Understanding by design* (2nd ed.). Association for Supervision and Curriculum Development.

# Worksheet 2-1:
# Teaching and Learning

As you consider the taxonomies of learning, which facilitates your thinking about your role as a clinical educator?

What are your goals or learning objectives for clinical education with those you work with?

## Backward Design for Clinical Education

What *results* do you want to see for the novice clinician you work with?

| Need to *know well*: | Need to *know and do*: | Need to *be familiar with*: |
|---|---|---|
|  |  |  |
|  |  |  |
|  |  |  |

| *Evidence* you will look for that will tell you the *results* have been achieved. | *Plan for learning and instruction* that will achieve the desired *results*. |
|---|---|
|  |  |
|  |  |
|  |  |

*(continued)*

# Worksheet 2-1:
# Teaching and Learning (continued)

**Reflections and Questions**

As you consider the learning objectives, learning taxonomies, and design for clinical education, give yourself a chance to reflect:

| What questions do you have? (These may or may not repeat from Chapter 1 worksheet.) | What aspects of the process do you want to learn more about? | Are there aspects of teaching and learning that you have an interest in researching based on what you have learned so far? |
|---|---|---|
|  |  |  |
|  |  |  |
|  |  |  |

# Evidence-Based Practice and Clinical Education

*Carol C. Dudding, PhD, CCC-SLP, F-ASHA*

*It ain't what they call you, it's what you answer to.*
                                                    —W. C. Fields

Experienced clinical educators are quick to tell you how clinical education has changed over the years. Like fabled stories of how we scored assessments manually without the use of a computer, clinical educators will share stories of sitting in dark cramped spaces behind a two-way mirror observing novice clinicians enter the world of clinical practice. You may sense a bit of nostalgia for the "good old days" when a clinical educator was viewed as a wise guide who was to be admired and emulated. Like most reflections on the good old days, our memories are flawed. Never has our role in the education of new professionals been just about passing along clinical skills and creating others just like us. At least, that's not the whole story.

Whether formally or informally, clinical educators are engaged in so much more than observation. An effective clinical educator is all at once engaged in teaching, evaluation and assessment, service delivery, and supervision. Our teaching goes beyond direct instruction in the clinical skills

necessary for professional practice. Clinical educators are continually assessing both client and student outcomes to assure a balance of responsibility to clinical training and service delivery. They serve as advisors and mentors modeling ethical practices while balancing the needs of clients and students. Clinical educators are expected to foster clinical decision making in students while modeling professional behaviors by their own actions.

An increased awareness of the roles and responsibilities of those engaged in clinical education of students is what led to the change in name from the more generic terms supervisor and preceptor to the more specific reference as a *clinical educator*. A clinical educator refers to those engaged in the education of students enrolled in professional education programs. Clinical educators, therefore, can be clinical faculty employed at a college or university, as well as community-based practitioners who provide clinical education to students within their employment setting. Clinical educators across professions share a common goal to develop clinical and professional knowledge and skills for entry-level practice (Dudding et al., 2017).

DeRuiter, M., & Ginsberg, S. M. (Eds.). *Clinician's Guide to Applying, Conducting, and Disseminating Clinical Education Research* (pp. 21-31).

# A Brief History of Clinical Education

While clinical supervision has likely existed since ancient times, the historical record begins with early accounts of supervision occurring in the 18th and 19th centuries as part of the origins of social work and nursing (Milne, 2009; White & Winstanley, 2014). In the 1930s and 1940s, clinical supervision became an integral part of the education of health care professionals across disciplines such as nursing, medicine, psychology, and counseling (White & Winstanley, 2014). The 1970s and 1980s saw the emergence of research on supervision in which researchers began to identify the specific skill sets necessary for effective supervision (Anderson, 1988; Ellis, 2010; Goodyear & Bernard, 1998; Ladany et al., 1996; Milne, 2009; Stace & Drexler, 1969).

It followed that organizations such as the American Speech-Language-Hearing Association (ASHA) and the American Psychological Association (APA) began publishing position statements and guidelines specific to clinical supervision. These types of publications legitimized supervision as a distinct area of expertise and practice and stipulated that special preparation and training was needed to enable individuals to function competently as supervisors.

# Clinical Education as a Distinct Area of Practice

In reflecting on your own supervisory experiences as a student or new professional, you may have come to realize that even the most skilled clinicians may fall short in their ability to serve as effective clinical educators. Some clinicians–turned–clinical educators rely heavily on observation and modeling as a method of instruction. That is, they ask the novice clinician to observe them in practice and then carry out services in much the same manner. Other clinical educators ascribe to the "sink or swim" method and expect students to learn by trial and error. These shortcomings aren't necessarily due to a lack of motivation or interest, it may be that the experienced clinician is lacking the distinct knowledge and skills necessary for effective clinical education.

Presently, accreditation and certification bodies in nursing, medicine, psychology, and associated health care professions recognize clinical education and supervision as a distinct area of practice requiring a specific set of knowledge and skills. Perhaps no group has more strongly advocated for the recognition of clinical supervision than the APA (2014):

Supervision is a distinct professional practice employing a collaborative relationship that has both facilitative and evaluative components, that extends over time, which has the goals of enhancing the professional competence and science-informed practice of the supervisee, monitoring the quality of services provided, protecting the public, and providing a gatekeeping function for entry into the profession. (p. 2)

# Knowledge, Skills, and Attitudes in Clinical Education

Researchers across health care disciplines have identified knowledge, skills, and attitudes necessary for effective clinical education. The APA has a long history of focus and research in the area of clinical supervision. They have developed seven domains that encompass specific knowledge, skills, and attitudes to achieve competency in clinical supervision that can readily be applied to other disciplines engaged in clinical education (APA, 2014). Some domains relate to the training and ethical and professional behaviors required of the clinical educator. Other domains focus on the supervisory relationship and methods of evaluation, assessment, and feedback. Those interested in a more detailed examination of these knowledge and skills should refer to Table 3-1.

# Training Requirements

It follows that with the recognition of clinical education as a distinct area of practice, and the establishment of knowledge, skills, and attitudes specific to supervision, organizations would require training for those engaged in clinical supervision. For example, the Council of Academic Programs in Communication Sciences and Disorders published a white paper recommending training for those engaged in clinical education in speech-language pathology and audiology (2013). In 2016, ASHA's Ad Hoc Committee on Supervisory Training recommended a minimum of 2 hours of professional development in supervision training for members engaged in clinical education of students and mentoring of clinical fellows (ASHA, 2016). This same committee put forth a rubric for self-assessment in supervision competencies that may be helpful to the reader in determining areas for training. See Table 3-2 for a listing of practice guidelines and training requirements for clinical education by professional organization.

**Table 3-1**

## American Psychological Association Competency-Based Domains of Clinical Supervision

| DOMAIN | COMPETENCY |
|---|---|
| Supervisor competence | The supervisor serves as a role model for the supervisee, fulfills the highest duty of protecting the public, and is a gatekeeper for the profession ensuring that supervisees meet competence standards in order to advance to the next level or to licensure. |
| Diversity | The supervisor infuses diversity into all aspects of clinical practice and supervision, including attention to oppression and privilege and the impact of those on the supervisory power differential, relationship, and on client/patient and supervisee interactions and supervision interactions. |
| Supervisory relationship | The supervisor bears responsibility for managing, collaborating, and discussing power within the relationship. |
| Professionalism | The supervisor reflects the essential professional characteristics of integrity, honesty, personal responsibility, and adherence to professional values, deportment, accountability, concern for the welfare of others, and professional identity. |
| Assessment, evaluation, and feedback | The supervisor provides timely assessment, evaluation, and feedback that is directly linked to specific competencies and observed behaviors. |
| Professional competence problems | The supervisor must protect the well-being of clients/patients and the general public while simultaneously supporting the professional development of the supervisee. |
| Ethical, legal, and regulatory considerations | The supervisor models ethical behavior, and adherence to relevant legal and regulatory parameters in supervision is essential to upholding the highest duty of the supervisor, protecting the public. |

Reproduced with permission from Board of Educational Affairs Task Force on Supervision Guidelines. (2014). *APA guidelines for clinical supervision in health service psychology* (pp. 9-20). American Psychological Association. https://www.apa.org/about/policy/guidelines-supervision.pdf. No further reproduction or distribution is permitted.

Those interested in advancing their knowledge and understanding of the evidence-based practices (EBPs) in clinical education are encouraged to seek training that goes beyond the minimum requirements put forth by professional organizations. Opportunities for training in supervision can be accessed through your own professional organization as well as other organizations with a shared investment in supervision (e.g., National Board of Certified Counselors, Council on Social Work Education, APA). The organizations referenced in Table 3-2 are a good starting place for those seeking advanced training in supervision.

Some clinical educators are surprised to learn there are organizations, journals, and special interest groups outside of their discipline-specific organizations dedicated to the dissemination of research related to evidence-based education-clinical education (EBE-CE). Table 3-3 offers a partial listing of these constituent groups, journals, and web-based resources. This information may serve as a starting point for those new to EBE-CE. For others, it may help you identify venues for publication of your research in this important area of study.

Those who have dedicated their careers to clinical education of future professionals have long advocated for specialty recognition in this distinct area of practice. Currently organizations such as the Accreditation Commission for Education in Nursing, the Accreditation Council for Occupational Therapy Education, and the National Board for Certified Counselors, offer special recognition in supervision and clinical education.

## Factors Impacting Clinical Education

It is important to be aware of the factors that impact our professional careers. Those who currently identify as clinical educators have likely been faced with challenges and changes impacting the training of students. It is important that we are aware of these factors so we can change and adjust our training practices to continue to train competent professionals able to meet the changing needs of our professions. It is also important that we consider how these factors impact how we apply, conduct, and disseminate research in clinical education.

The rapid changes and advancement in health care practices is undeniable. Advances in technology and interprofessional practice (IPP) have significantly improved patient outcomes. The changes have resulted in changes in the nature and diversity of client caseloads, expanding scopes of practice, and a mandate to prepare students ready to enter a complex workforce. The improvements in health care

**Table 3-2**

## PRACTICE AND TRAINING REQUIREMENT OF PROFESSIONAL ORGANIZATIONS

| ORGANIZATIONAL BODY | GUIDING DOCUMENTS | SUPERVISORY TRAINING REQUIREMENTS BEYOND PROFESSIONAL LICENSURE AND CREDENTIALING |
|---|---|---|
| Accreditation Commission for Education in Nursing https://www.acenursing.org | Accreditation Commission for Education in Nursing Accreditation Manual 2017 Standards and Criteria https://www.acenursing.org/acen-accreditation-manual/ | |
| Accreditation Council for Graduate Medical Education | Accreditation Council for Graduate Medical Education Common Program Requirements (Residency) https://www.acgme.org/globalassets/PFAssets/ProgramRequirements/CPRResidency_2022v2.pdf | |
| Accreditation Council for Occupational Therapy Education https://acoteonline.org/all-schools/ | 2018 Accreditation Council for Occupational Therapy Education Standards and Interpretive Guide https://acoteonline.org/download/3751/ | |
| American Academy of Audiology | Clinical Education Guidelines for Audiology Externships https://www.audiology.org/wp-content/uploads/2021/05/Clinical-Education-Guidelines-for-Audiology-Externships.pdf | |
| American Association of Colleges of Nursing https://www.aacnnursing.org/CCNE | Standards for Accreditation of Baccalaureate and Graduate Nursing Programs https://www.aacnnursing.org/Portals/42/CCNE/PDF/Standards-Final-2018.pdf | |
| APA | Guidelines for Clinical Supervision in Health Service Psychology https://www.apa.org/about/policy/guidelines-supervision.pdf | Varies by state licensing board |
| ASHA (Council for Clinical Certification) | Knowledge and Skills Needed by Speech-Language Pathologists Providing Clinical Supervision https://www.asha.org/policy/ks2008-00294/ | 2 hours minimum post-certification when supervising students and/or mentoring clinical fellows |
| Commission on Accreditation in Physical Therapy Education | Standards and Required Elements for Accreditation of Physical Therapist Education Programs https://www.capteonline.org/globalassets/capte-docs/capte-pt-standards-required-elements.pdf | |
| Council on Social Work Education https://www.cswe.org/#:~:text=CSWE's%20Commission%20on%20Accreditation%20is,United%20States%20and%20its%20territories | 2015 Educational Policy and Accreditation Standards https://www.cswe.org/accreditation/policies-process/2022epas/ | Varies by state licensing board |
| National Board for Certified Counselors | Approved Clinical Supervisor Credential Eligibility Policy https://www.cce-global.org/Assets/ACS/ACS_Eligibility_Policy.pdf | 45 hours of clinical supervision training, or 3-semester-hour graduate course or an equivalent course from a Council for Accreditation of Counseling and Related Educational Programs accredited program No exam required |

## Table 3-3

### RESOURCES DEDICATED TO EVIDENCE-BASED EDUCATION-CLINICAL EDUCATION

| DOMAIN | COMPETENCY |
|---|---|
| Journals | *ASHA Perspectives Administration and Supervision* |
| | *Counselor Education and Supervision* |
| | *Journal of Counselor Preparation and Supervision* |
| | *Journal of Educational Supervision* |
| | *Journal of Social Work Education* |
| | *Journal of Sports Administration & Supervision* |
| | *Scholarship of Teaching and Learning in Psychology* |
| | *Teaching and Learning in Communication Sciences & Disorders* |
| | *Teaching and Supervision in Counseling* |
| | *The Clinical Supervisor* |
| Special interest groups/divisions | ASHA Special Interest Group 11 Administration and Supervision |
| | National Consortium of Clinical Educators |
| | Southeastern University Clinical Educators Network |
| Training opportunities | American Occupational Therapy Association Fieldwork Educators Certificate Program |
| | Council of Academic Programs in Communication Sciences and Disorders eLearning Modules |
| | Harvard Medical School Training to Teach in Medicine certificate |
| | National League for Nursing Certification for Nurse Educators |
| | National Association of Social Workers clinical supervision courses |
| | Preceptor Education Program |
| Web-based resources | ASHA Clinical Education and Supervision Practice Portal |
| | Nursing Education Network |

---

## BOX 3-1:
### FACTORS IMPACTING CLINICAL EDUCATION

- Expanding scope of practice
- Changes in accreditation and certification standards
- Increasing demands of workplace settings
- Call for interprofessional education (IPE)/collaborative practice
- Use of technology for student training and service delivery
- Increased student diversity
- Emerging recognition of implicit and explicit biases
- Scarcity of external clinical placements
- Decreased funding to higher education
- Increased focus on EBPs

---

and neurodiversity—those individuals who have survived strokes, devastating brain injuries, childhood injuries, and cancer. As survival rates for children born prematurely increase, so does the need to be able to competently evaluate and treat these children in school-based settings. These changes in clinical practice require an expanding scope of practice, which in turn, requires an expansion of the standards and credentials that govern our professions.

The expanding scope of practice in our professional work settings and changes in practice standards have a direct impact on what, when, how, and where we train our students. One such change is related to the rapid expansion and sophistication of technologies employed in the medical and educational settings. Programs need to be able to offer students training and hands-on experiences with a widening range of technologies found in practice settings. It can be challenging for a university program to secure all models of digital hearing aids and the accompanying software for their students' practice. It is equally challenging to offer students a well-resourced lab with all the latest augmentative and alternative communication devices. Not only is this a drain on financial resources and space, but it also puts a strain on the clinical educators directly involved in student training and education. Novice clinicians in psychology

outcomes for all of us has changed the very nature of those we serve on our caseloads. As practitioners, we must now be prepared to work with persons with brain differences

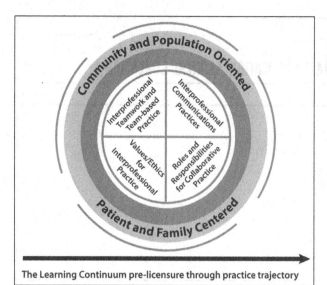

**Figure 3-1.** Interprofessional Education Collaborative competencies for interprofessional collaborative practice. (Reproduced with permission from Interprofessional Education Collaborative. [2016]. *Core competencies for interprofessional collaborative practice: 2016 update.* Author.)

must learn not only how to conduct neuropsychological testing instruments. In medicine, they need to gain hands-on experience with ultrasound technology. And, of course, virtually all clinicians need experience learning how to use electronic medical records and providing services through telehealth. Clinical educators find themselves challenged by the time and expertise needed to stay current on all the demands of the workplaces in which our students find themselves.

## Interprofessional Education

Another area that has significance for clinical education is IPE. IPE is the companion to IPP. IPP has been shown to contribute to improved outcomes in health care. It is recognized that training programs need to provide students with the competencies in order to practice in a collaborative and interprofessional workplace. In 2003, the Institute of Medicine determined core competencies for IPE. Since that time, most professional organizations have adopted the four core competencies developed by the Interprofessional Education Collaborative (2016). College and university training programs must commit to training future health care professionals in how to practice in the interprofessional environment for IPP to reach its full potential. Figure 3-1 is a commonly used representation of the Interprofessional Education Collaborative competencies for interprofessional collaborative practice.

## Changes in Student Demographics

Changes in the demographics of our students is another area for consideration. Graduate training programs are experiencing a more diverse student body in terms of an increase of diversity in age, gender, culture, and experiences. Professional programs nationwide are called to do better in attracting and maintaining racially diverse people to our programs. Diversity of all types is highly desirable and key to the health of our professions. It is often the case that clinical educators and students are of different backgrounds and experiences, resulting in implicit and explicit biases within the clinical education process. These biases need to be better studied to address disservice to our underrepresented student groups. It is also incumbent upon us as clinical educators to better prepare future professionals to fairly and justly provide services to an increasingly diverse client/patient population.

## Other Challenges

The interrelationships between clinical education programs and professional settings is a key factor affecting the professions. Many programs in higher education across professions, such as nursing, social work, physical therapy, occupational therapy, and speech-language pathology, report a scarcity of external clinical placements for our students. While this is a complex issue, increased demands for productivity in the workplace, a lack of adequate compensation and/or recognition for their service as clinical educators, time-consuming and resource-intensive processes, and a perceived disconnect between the practice settings and university (Taylor et al., 2017) are all factors to be considered.

Further complicating the issues, institutions of higher education are dealing with declining enrollments, decreased public funding, and shortages of qualified faculty. That means that faculty, including clinical educators, are being asked to do more with less. The COVID-19 global pandemic has put additional stress and strains on clinical placements in ways that are still unknown. What is known is that changes in workplace settings and stressors in higher education will have a significant impact on clinical education programs.

It is not the intent of this chapter to argue the importance of clinical education in the training of future professionals. Its purpose is to provide you with some background and history to provide you with a context in which to consider your role as a clinical educator. Moving forward, you will be directed to current EBPs in supervision and clinical education. From there you will consider the importance of research in clinical education, as well as your role in that process. The desired outcome is that you will finish this chapter with a head full of questions and a strong desire to seek answers for a select few of them.

# MODELS OF CLINICAL EDUCATION

There are a number of long-standing, as well as newer, emerging models of supervision to consider within the context of clinical education of students. These models tend to take on the underpinnings of the discipline that first created the approach. That is, psychology and counseling may take on more of a psychoanalytical approach to clinical supervision, whereas other disciplines may be more focused on specific knowledge and skills.

Models of supervision may be categorized into several categories for purposes of discussion:

- Developmental/continuum models
- Cognitive-apprenticeship models
- Competency-based models
- Placement models (Adapted from Leddick, 1994; Wolford et al., 2021)

## Developmental/Continuum Models

Developmental models of supervision hold the premise that supervisees move through somewhat predictable stages of growth and development on the path to becoming independent professionals. Developmental models often use labels such as novice, intermediate, and advanced when categorizing students. Novice or entry-level students often are highly motivated, yet report high anxiety and fear of evaluation (Stoltenberg et al., 1998). They are likely to require more direct forms of supervision and require a good deal of feedback. Mid-level students experience fluctuating confidence and motivation, and advanced students are said to be stable in motivation and objectivity (Stoltenberg et al., 1998), requiring a less direct input from the supervisor. Within these models, the behavior of the supervisor changes in response to the needs of the supervisee. For example, Anderson's Continuum of Supervision (Anderson, 1988) clearly describes how the supervisor moves from a direct-active style toward a collaborative approach as the student assumes more responsibility and independence.

## Cognitive-Apprenticeship Models

Cognitive-apprenticeship models of supervision, as the name implies, rely on the development of cognitive practices that lead to the learning of complex processes (Stalmeijer, 2015). The four domains include acquiring content knowledge, apprenticeship training, sequencing, and situated learning. The supervisor employs modeling, coaching, and scaffolding to guide the student in guided practice. While this model was first employed in the training of psychotherapy, the techniques of modeling,

coaching, and scaffolding can be applied to many clinical supervision models. Additionally, the use of Socratic questioning, reflection, and exploration on the part of the student helps to make the clinical decision making more explicit. Apprenticeship training is an aspect of training that is familiar to many students in the health care arena. This model is often implemented as a 1:1 relationship between a supervisor and supervisee.

## Competency-Based Models

There is an emerging interest in competency-based models of supervision across disciplines nationally and internationally (Gonsalvez & Calvert, 2014). Competency-based models have as their goal the making of a competent professional. Professional competence in this sense is more than an expansive checklist of knowledge and skills. Professional competence encompasses higher order thinking, judgment, reasoning skills, and behaviors across domains (Gonsalvez & Calvert, 2014). Competency-based models of supervision are focused on the output (e.g., student outcomes) and don't rely on the input (e.g., completion of a certain number of clinical clock hours) to determine competency. Competency-based models are readily integrated into other models of supervision. Competency-based models of supervision are easily aligned with EBP and EBP-CE.

## Placement Models

The supervisory models previously discussed occur in varying contexts and across settings. It is common practice for students to obtain clinical training in university clinics, externships, and internships. Traditionally, students are placed with a single supervisor for a specified period of time (e.g., one semester). Yet, there are other models to be considered. Sheepway and colleagues (2011) described various models in terms of types of supervision, student-to-supervisor ratio and mode of supervision. As mentioned, the 1:1 supervisor to student ratio is commonly found as part of the apprenticeship model. Researchers are exploring alternative models, such as 2:1 ratio (two students and one supervisor), group supervision (two or more students with two or more supervisors), and shared supervision (one student with more than one supervisor). The qualifications of the supervisor is often determined by the standards of the organizations, but in some cases, professionals outside of the discipline are permitted to serve as supervisors. That is particularly the case in interprofessional settings where students participate in shared learning experiences supervised by a number of professionals.

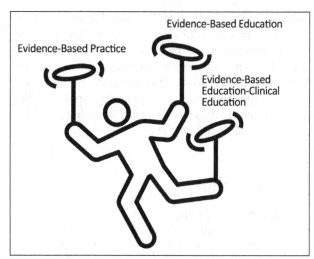

**Figure 3-2.** Juggling EBP and EBE in clinical education.

# EVIDENCE-BASED PRACTICE IN CLINICAL EDUCATION

We began this chapter by describing the many roles of the clinical educator being teaching, evaluation and assessment, service delivery, and supervision. You may find yourself at times juggling the demands of these roles. Clinical educators are further called upon to juggle the demands of both EBP and EBE, as conceptualized in Figure 3-2. EBP is a standard of care that requires the clinician to apply or translate research findings in clinical practices and clinical decision making. EBP is determined by a combination of best evidence, patient wants and needs, and a practitioner's clinical knowledge and skills. EBE is based on the principle that educational practices should be based on evidence and not tradition. Like EPB, EBE is multifaceted. EBE requires the educator to consider best evidence in teaching and learning, the experiences and needs of the learners, and their own knowledge and skills in teaching when determining the best approach to education (Davies, 1999). DeRuiter and Ginsberg (2020) refer to this as the EBE-CE model in recognition of the unique responsibility that clinical educators have in shifting and combining both EBP and EPE as part of clinical education models.

So why is it important for us as clinical educators to engage in this discussion about EBE-CE? A conscious and deliberate approach to EBE-CE has the benefit of:

- Heightening reflection on practice
- Improving reliance on the existing and evolving body of evidence
- Shaping the future of ongoing research into the clinical education
- Improving our knowledge base (DeRuiter & Ginsberg, 2020)

## Importance of Research in Clinical Education

As we begin to examine EBE as it applies to clinical education, it is imperative that we do so from a solid knowledge base. However, we soon realize that there is a small but emerging body of evidence as to what makes up EBPs in clinical education. The remainder of this workbook will provide you with detailed descriptions of how to go about applying, conducting, and disseminating research in this area. These lessons apply whether you intend to conduct and publish your own original research or are a dedicated clinical educator interested in investigating and evaluating your own clinical education practice.

The good news is that we are not alone in the commitment to research specific to EBE-CE. In 1998, a dedicated and passionate group of international educators rang the alarm about the lack of scholarly research in clinical education of doctors (Harden et al., 1999; Hart & Harden, 2000). An article appeared in the *British Medical Journal* with the clear call to action: "The evidence-base is as important in educating new doctors as it is in assessing a new chemotherapy" (Petersen, 1999, p. 1223). Embedded in this argument is the claim that improved educational training is essential in producing better doctors, which leads to improved medical outcomes (Harden et al., 1999). This argument is easily translated to the training of health care professionals in other disciplines of study.

These educators did not stop there. This call to action led to the creation of an international organization called the Best Evidence Medical and Health Professional Education (BEME) Collaboration. The BEME Collaboration is made up of individuals, medical universities, and professional organizations committed to the development of evidence-informed education in the medical and health professions. The BEME Collaborative has published a series of BEME Guides developed to advance EBE. Topics include how to conduct systematic reviews of existing evidence, the use of simulations for clinical teaching, evidence related to the use of assessment and feedback in clinical education, and learning outcomes as predictors of success. Those interested can access BEME and other resources, including the guides and also podcasts, by visiting the International Association for Health Professions Education at https://amee.org/.

## An Approach to Evidence-Based Clinical Education

Before moving forward in our quest for EBE-CE, it might be helpful to consider the steps in EBE-CE. Figure 3-3 offers a five-step approach. The steps begin with framing the question, gathering the evidence, evaluating the evidence, implementing change based on the evidence, and evaluating the resulting outcomes. This approach is based

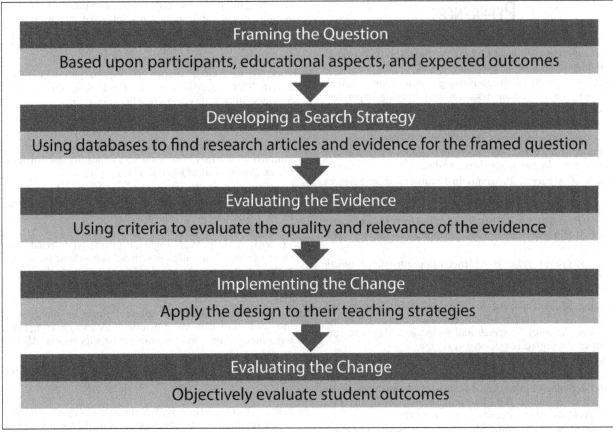

**Figure 3-3.** Steps in evidence-based clinical education. Based on the BEME model. (Adapted from Harden, R. M., Grant, J., Buckley, G., & Hart, I. R. [1999]. BEME Guide No. 1: Best evidence medical education. *Medical Teacher, 21*[6], 553-562. https://doi.org/10.1080/01421599978960 and Masoomi, R. [2012]. What is the best evidence medical education? *Research and Development in Medical Education, 1*[1], 3-5. https://doi.org/10.5681/rdme.2012.002)

on the BEME model developed by Harden and colleagues (1999) and follows other approaches to EBPs. See Chapter 4 for a detailed account of the steps involved in EBE-CE.

The very fact that you have chosen to read this text means that you are interested in the research evidence, either as a consumer or producer of research. In either scenario, your interest is likely inspired by a need in the form of a question. For example, why do some students struggle with making appropriate referrals? What is the best way to help students apply the knowledge acquired in the classroom to the clinical setting? Are simulations worth the time and money? What are the systemic biases in the current system that affect students of color? The depth and breadth of these questions is only limited by the number of clinical educators engaged in the research process.

# Summary

Going back to the quote at the very beginning of this chapter, "It ain't what they call you, it's what you answer to," attributed to W. C. Fields. Whether you are called a supervisor, preceptor, or clinical educator, you are above all an educator. Whether you are called a clinician, therapist, or researcher, you are above all an educator. You are an educator with an awesome responsibility to guide, teach, and inspire the next generation of practitioners. Your role goes well beyond the teaching of skills and transferring of knowledge. Your role is to serve as a role model, engage in a supervisory relationship that values diversity and provides a safe environment for learning, conduct yourself with personal and professional integrity, while simultaneously protecting the public and those that we professionally serve.

By systematically engaging with the research, you are ensuring that your clinical education practices are informed by a research base. You are engaging in professional development that not only benefits you but those that you educate. By actively engaging with the research, you are instilling the qualities of life-long learning in your students. By purposefully engaging with the research, you are positively impacting the future of your students, their clients, and the profession to which you belong.

# REFERENCES

American Psychological Association. (2014). *Guidelines for clinical supervision in health service psychology.* http://apa.org/about/policy/guidelines-supervision.pdf

American Speech-Language-Hearing Association. (2016). *A plan for developing resources and training opportunities in clinical supervision* [Final report of ASHA Ad Hoc Committee on Supervision Training]. https://www.asha.org/siteassets/reports/ahc-on-supervision-training.pdf

Anderson, J. L. (1988). *The supervisory process in speech language pathology and audiology.* Pro-Ed.

Council of Academic Programs in Communication Sciences and Disorders. (2013). *White paper: Preparation of speech-language pathology clinical educators.* http://scotthall.dotster.com/capcsd/wp-content/uploads/2014/10/Preparation-of-Clinical-Educators-White-Paper.pdf

Davies, P. (1999). What is evidence-based education? *British Journal of Educational Studies, 47*(2), 108-121. [Taylor & Francis Online].

DeRuiter, M., & Ginsberg, S. M. (2020). Conscious clinical education: The evidence-based education-clinical education model. *Seminars in Speech and Language, 41*(4), 279-288, https://doi.org/10.1055/s-0040-1713779

Dudding, C. C., McCready, V., Nunez, L. M., & Procaccini, S. J. (2017). Clinical supervision in speech-language pathology and audiology in the United States: Development of a professional specialty. *The Clinical Supervisor, 36*(2), 161-181. https://doi.org/10.1080/07325223.2017.1377663

Ellis, M. V. (2010). Bridging the science and practice of clinical supervision: Some discoveries, some misconceptions. *The Clinical Supervisor, 29*(1), 95-116. https://doi.org/10.1080/07325221003741910

Gonsalvez, C., & Calvert, F. L. (2014). Competency-based models of supervision: Principles and applications, promises and challenges. *Australian Psychologist, 49*(4), 200-208. https://doi.org/10.1111/AP.12055

Goodyear, R. K., & Bernard, J. M. (1998). Clinical supervision: Lessons from the literature. *Counselor Education & Supervision, 38,* 6-22.

Harden, R. M., Grant, J., Buckley, G., & Hart, I. R. (1999). BEME Guide No. 1: Best evidence medical education. *Medical Teacher, 21*(6), 553-562. https://doi.org/10.1080/01421599978960

Hart, I. R., & Harden, R. M. (2000). Best evidence medical education (BEME): A plan for action. *Medical Teacher, 22*(2), 131-135. https://doi.org/10.1080/01421590078535

Interprofessional Education Collaborative. (2016). *Core competencies for interprofessional collaborative practice: 2016 update.* Author.

Ladany, N., Hill, C. E., Corbett, M. M., & Nutt, E. A. (1996). Nature, extent, and importance of what psychotherapy trainees do not disclose to their supervisors. *Journal of Counseling Psychology, 43*(1), 10-24. https://doi.org/10.1037/0022-0167.43.1.10

Leddick, G. R. (1994). *Models of clinical supervision. ERIC Digest.* ERIC Clearinghouse on Counseling and Student Services. https://eric.ed.gov/?id=ED372340

Milne, D. (2009). *Evidence-based clinical supervision: Principles and practice* (pp. xi, 272). British Psychological Society.

Petersen, S. (1999). Time for evidence based medical education: Tomorrow's doctors need informed educators not amateur tutors. *British Medical Journal, 318,* 1223-1224.

Rotgans, J. I. (2012). The themes, institutions, and people of medical education research 1988-2010: Content analysis of abstracts from six journals. *Advances in Health Sciences Education, 17,* 515-527.

Sheepway, L., Lincoln, M., & Togher, L. (2011). An international study of clinical education practices in speech-language pathology. *International Journal of Speech-Language Pathology, 13*(2), 174-185. https://doi.org/10.3109/17549507.2011.491129

Stace, A., & Drexler, A. (1969). Special training for supervisors of student clinicians: What private speech and hearing centers do and think about training their supervisors. *ASHA, 11,* 318-320.

Stalmeijer, R. E. (2015). When I say … cognitive apprenticeship. *Medical Education, 49*(4), 355-356. https://doi.org/10.1111/medu.12630

Stoltenberg, C. D., McNeill, B., & Delworth, U. (1998). *IDM supervision: An integrated developmental model for supervising counselors and therapists.* Jossey Bass.

Taylor, C., Angel, L., Nyanga, L., & Dickson, C. (2017). The process and challenges of obtaining and sustaining clinical placements for nursing and allied health students. *Journal of Clinical Nursing, 26*(19-20), 3099-3110. https://doi.org/10.1111/jocn.13658

White, E., & Winstanley, J. (2014). Clinical supervision and the helping professions: An interpretation of history. *The Clinical Supervisor, 33*(1), 3-25. https://doi.org/10.1080/07325223.2014.905226

Wolford, G. L., Wolford, L., Fissel Brannick, S., Scott, M., & Smith, R. (2021). "Shouldn't you be collaborative by now?": Supervisory needs, expectations, and satisfaction across the educational trajectory in speech-language pathology. *The Clinical Supervisor, 40*(2), 241-262. https://doi.org/10.1080/07325223.2020.1833268

# Worksheet 3-1:
# Evidence-Based Practice in Clinical Education

**Potential Research Topics in Clinical Education**

| EBE-CE Area | Clinical Education Research Topic (Rotgans, 2012) |
|---|---|
| Expanding scope of practice | Student assessment and evaluation |
| Changes in accreditation and certification standards | Use of simulations in clinical skills training |
| Increasing demands of workplace settings | Models of supervision |
| Call for IPE/collaborative practice | Problem-based learning |
| Use of technology for student training and service delivery | Community-based training |
| | Clinical competence assessment |
| Increased student diversity | Student characteristics |
| Emerging recognition of implicit and explicit biases | IPE |
| Scarcity of external clinical placements | Clinical reasoning and decision making |
| Increased focus on EBPs | Attitudes, cultural competence, ethics |
| | Underrepresented minority students |
| | Costs of health care education |
| | Computer-assisted instruction |
| | Faculty development and training |

**Reflections and Questions**

As you consider the wide range of aspects of our field, including changing practice models, practice settings, and widening scope of practice, do you find your questions evolving, becoming more specific, or different?

# Research as Professional Development for Clinical Educators

*Sarah M. Ginsberg, EdD, CCC-SLP, F-ASHA*
*and Mark DeRuiter, MBA, PhD, CCC-A/SLP, F-ASHA*

In Chapter 1, we talked briefly about our struggles to figure out our professional identities in the push and pull between clinical work and educational work. For many of us, the process of initially finishing our education meant that we began working in our discipline as clinicians in some clinical setting. At that stage, we saw ourselves as clinicians and sought out professional development opportunities for clinically oriented challenges we were facing in the workplace or for skills we wanted to acquire. Fast forward to engaging in education, in the classroom or the clinical setting or both, and you might have found yourself questioning your professional identity in regards to clinician or educator, or both. When I (SMG) was at the earliest stages of working in academia, I not only found myself wondering if I was a clinician or an educator, I found myself feeling pulled in terms of professional development materials. Should I learn more about the patients that I was treating, or should I learn about how to teach a course on the disorders that I was teaching or how to supervise students conducting evaluations in the university clinic where I was a clinical educator? For quite a while I was juggling the roles of clinician, clinical educator, and academic educator simultaneously. It felt like there was not enough time to learn everything I wanted to know through professional development.

## PROFESSIONAL DEVELOPMENT

For many professionals in health care, the concept of continuing education or professional development became a requirement for practice sometime in the 20th century. Medicine began requiring continuing education in the 1960s (Institute of Medicine, 2010). Formal continuing education in nursing began appearing in the middle of the 20th century as well (Stein, 2021). Physical therapy and speech-language pathology began requiring continuing education toward the latter half of the 20th century. Known by various terms, including professional development, continuing education, and continuing professional development, the purpose of professional development, which will be used as an umbrella term for our discussion here, is to enhance and expand our knowledge and skills for professional practice (Filipe et al., 2014; Traylor et al., 2020).

The challenge for those of us playing multiple roles in our profession is that there may be numerous aspects of knowledge and skills that need to be addressed by the multiple roles that we play. In the ideal world, professionals have time to reflect on their "learning need" (Filipe et

DeRuiter, M., & Ginsberg, S. M. (Eds.). *Clinician's Guide to Applying,*
*Conducting, and Disseminating Clinical Education Research* (pp. 33-48).

al., 2014, p. 138), which is defined as the "gap" (Filipe et al., 2014, p. 138) between current knowledge and competencies and the knowledge and skills that would allow a professional to support their effective practice for whatever role they play. This may include clinical care, organizational management, clinical education, and research (Roberts et al., 2014; Traylor et al., 2020). There are a number of challenges that we are all likely to face in trying to complete professional development for even our primary role. When we add multiple roles that would benefit from professional development, the challenges may feel insurmountable. Some common barriers to completion of professional development may include:

- Time constraints
- Time available in your own day-to-day life
- Time not allocated by your employer
- Financial limitations
- Out-of-pocket expenses
- Employer does not fund professional development
- Awareness of professional development opportunities
- Unfamiliar with how to access resources
- Unaware of materials or programs that would support specific goals

The last barrier of being unaware that materials are available to support specific goals can be particularly difficult. If you have not come to think of yourself as a clinical educator—*I'm just a clinician that my director asked to supervise a university student*—you might also not have had time to reflect on the fact that your professional roles are evolving, let alone consider that there may be resources available that would help you perform the role in a more effective, evidence-based manner. Life is busy, we don't always have the luxury to stop and think about how our scope of work is changing slowly over time and how to support ourselves with professional development.

# EVIDENCE-BASED PRACTICE PROFESSIONAL DEVELOPMENT

In Chapter 1, we introduced and reviewed the models of evidence-based practice (EBP), evidence-based education (EBE), and evidence-based education-clinical education (EBE-CE). Here we will connect those models to the ways we think about professional development to support us in those roles. Given that there may be significant challenges to professional development for a variety of our roles, let's take a minute to think about what the focus of professional development might be for each. In considering EBP, these aspects of our roles are the ones we are most familiar with, particularly when it comes to professional development. Most of us focus our professional development in this

domain on approaches to assessment of a disorder where the assessment approach is new or the disorder is one we have less experience with. We might be seeking out learning opportunities that help us improve the patients' outcomes or treatments that are more effective than what we have tried previously. Ultimately, many of us use professional development as a way to keep up with new technologies, new assessment and treatment approaches, and move away from outdated or poorly supported methods toward those that demonstrate the potential for improved patient outcomes.

While we might have to work a bit to find the best fit between the learning materials that are out there and the patients that we are serving, there is likely an abundance of options available as this clinical work is the focus of professional development for many of our professions.

# EVIDENCE-BASED EDUCATION PROFESSIONAL DEVELOPMENT

We can think about the key roles that EBE can play in higher education, helping us learn new and improved technologies and methodologies available to improve student outcomes. Much as we engage in professional development for EBP to improve patient outcomes, we want students to learn as effectively as possible such that they are successful clinicians. Many of us have memories of the way learning was structured for us when we were in school. As new educators, or educators who have not had a chance to engage in professional development for EBE, we may teach the way we were taught. It is familiar, it may seem the path of least resistance, or it is simple to organize teaching and learning in this way. We get it. And to be fair, many of us had instructors who were very effective with their teaching approaches more than 30 years ago before the idea of the scholarship of teaching and learning (SoTL) even became popular. We will shortly talk more about this later, but for now, consider that by engaging in professional development for EBE content, you may learn there are changes you can make to your teaching, no matter what setting you are in and no matter what content you are teaching, that might make your performance in this role even better. Your students might demonstrate better retention of the material, better application of the content, and you might improve not only their satisfaction with the educational experience but you might improve your own as well (Roberts et al., 2014).

## Within and Across Disciplines

As you look for professional development materials for EBE, you may find yourself seeking out content that is specific to your discipline, or you may find that related disciplines have content that is valuable for you to learn from. There are benefits to both. As a speech-language pathologist trying to improve my student's understanding of neuroanatomy, I might first seek out materials that address the teaching and learning process in my discipline: What research has been conducted to demonstrate the most effective manner of helping students learn neuroanatomy in a way that has the best results for clinical applications in speech-language pathology? However, just as we see in EBP and in finding literature about a variety of topics, we might find a gap in the literature that has not been filled within our discipline (see Chapter 8 for more information regarding finding the gap in literature). If I cannot find information within my own discipline, it might be useful to me to explore the literature in related disciplines, such as occupational therapy, physical therapy, or physician assistant education. If I learn of a method that has been demonstrated to be effective in teaching neuroanatomy in one of those fields, I might be able to adopt the technique for use in my own teaching context. In my experience, as an educator and as a clinician, I have found that I am able to learn and apply information that comes from fields other than my own. I would encourage you to explore beyond the boundaries of your own discipline and see what you can learn from colleagues in other disciplines.

## Evidence-Based Education-Clinical Education Professional Development

As we consider the EBE-CE model as a whole, we realize that in addition to needing professional development that focuses on EBP and EBE, we need to consider the role that we take as a clinical educator specifically into account by looking at the factors that also impact how we do our jobs. These include balancing our organizational needs, such as completing paperwork, maintaining productivity standards, and nurturing client relationships, even when we remove ourselves temporarily from the clinical process when our student clinician becomes the principal clinician for a period of time. We contend that the multifaceted nature of the work of a clinical educator—managing the outcomes and expectations of patients, students, and your job-related expectations—is one of the most demanding and complicated roles we can play (DeRuiter & Ginsberg, 2020). Additionally, we have previously acknowledged that the components within the middle aspect of the clinical education model are "hidden" because the factors are not always acknowledged and reflected upon by those engaged in doing this work (p. 282). And yet, it is often undervalued and undersupported, further complicating the ability to do the work well.

In many fields, professional development for the role of clinical educator is the least abundant, in contrast to EBP and EBE. Topics that may be helpful in supporting your work in this role, in addition to what has already been described, may include research regarding the best mechanisms for mediating the student-client relationship, for assessing student outcomes that are consistent with your profession but also for your organization, and how to structure teaching and learning for novice clinicians in light of particularly challenging patients. In many clinical fields, this represents a relatively new line of work as the demands of juggling all parties' needs are just beginning to be fully appreciated. Areas to consider seeking out professional development content that will support this role, in addition to what has already been described, include the ethical duties associated with the clinical educator role, managing relationships with all constituents, work/role demands, examining the clinical procedures that are in place in your setting, and even assessment of student performance (DeRuiter & Ginsberg, 2020). Figure 4-1 is provided to you in this chapter as a reminder of the complex factors and relationships that are at play in the EBE-CE environment.

## Targeting the Right Level of Professional Development

As you have probably noticed, we see considerable value in reflecting on the various roles we are asked to perform and how they evolve over time. As noted, this can be particularly challenging for the clinical educator because the shift to playing the role can be one that you did not elect to play or you saw it as a one-time experience, not necessarily a permanent and ongoing role. The subtle job creep can add to the unconscious nature of the work that you are called up to do and the inability to give all the time, attention, and professional development effort that you might like. The fact that this is a common experience is part of what has shaped the work we have done in the area of clinical educator in the last few years. In addition to considering the content that you might want to focus your professional development on, we would like to draw your attention to where you are on the continuum of clinical educator development.

McKinney (2007) proposed a framework for skill development in classroom-based higher education, which can be applied to advance your knowledge and skills as an educator that we have applied to the clinical education process (DeRuiter & Ginsberg, 2020). We describe this as a model of professional development for EBE-CE that is hierarchical in nature and can be represented graphically

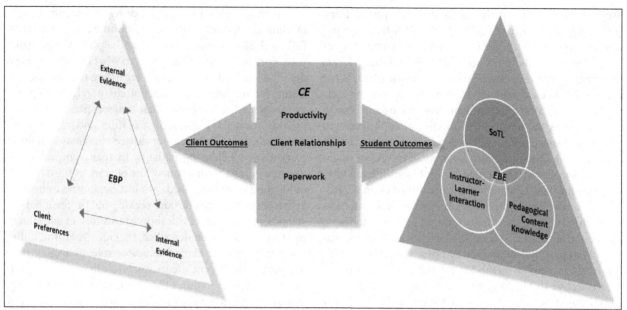

**Figure 4-1.** EBE-CE. (Reproduced with permission from DeRuiter, M., & Ginsberg, S. M. [2020]. Conscious clinical education: The evidence-based education-clinical education model. *Seminars in Speech and Language, 41*[4], 279-288. https://doi.org/10.1055/s-0040-1713779)

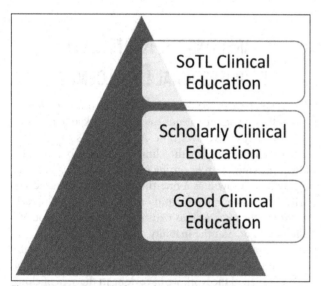

**Figure 4-2.** EBE-CE model for professional development. (Reproduced with permission from DeRuiter, M., & Ginsberg, S. M. [2020]. Conscious clinical education: The evidence-based education-clinical education model. *Seminars in Speech and Language, 41*[4], 279-288. https://doi.org/10.1055/s-0040-1713779)

(Figure 4-2). Considering the description of the levels of development and how they best fit may help guide you to move through the hierarchy and achieve the level of knowledge and skill that you are interested in for your clinical education work.

# Good Clinical Education

At the most fundamental level, clinical educators who consider through reflection, planning, and careful consideration the clinical education process are practicing *good clinical education*. It does not matter whether you are a full-time clinical educator working in a university clinic or are a clinical educator who is working with their first novice clinician in your clinical setting. If you have given thought as to how to help your student learn and become a good clinician, you are here. At the level of practicing good clinical education, you may be asking yourself about the process (DeRuiter & Ginsberg, 2020):

- Where do I begin structuring the learning process for this student?

- How do I approach the clinical educator process?

These questions may help you identify professional development that addresses your needs and level of learning most effectively. If a clinical educator is struggling with the novelty of the process or is supervising in a new context, they may also do well to consider the EBE-CE model to consciously reflect on the competing demands of their role and identify which aspects of evidence-based work present challenges.

# Scholarly Clinical Education

For some clinical educators, once they have gained some experience with the role or perform the role in more than one context, they begin to focus more specifically on further developing their own knowledge and skills as an educator. At this point, they may seek out the SoTL literature to learn more about what the evidence can tell us about the best ways to provide clinical education. The clinical educator is transitioning at this point to practicing *scholarly clinical education* (DeRuiter & Ginsberg, 2020). As noted before, SoTL research focuses on identifying best practices for education, including clinical education. Using the literature, in your field and related ones, can help you identify the most effective approaches to supervision in specific contexts, with particular types of students, or in evaluating and treating certain diagnoses. In effect, the clinical educator who is relying on the SoTL literature, as well as discussing challenges in clinical education with colleagues, and reflecting on how to best provide support to the novice clinicians using that information is taking the next step to become more evidence-based in their clinical education duties. As experienced clinical educators, we may be driven to the literature for the first time for a reason. We may have found ourselves struggling with how to help a student learn how to conduct an evaluation or perhaps they are frustrated that the feedback they are giving doesn't seem to be helping the student improve their skills. Clinical educators who have these thoughts may find themselves wondering:

- How can I obtain the best outcomes for my patient in the context of clinical education?
- What data exist for the methods I am using with the students in my clinic?
- Could we teach clinical writing in a way that creates efficiency in the process, thereby increasing the capacity for student education? (DeRuiter & Ginsberg, 2020, p. 286)

Asking more focused questions regarding what research has been done, in our own fields and related ones, will lead the scholarly clinical educator toward professional development opportunities that provide them with ideas for new and potentially more effective educational strategies that are evidence-based and can be adapted for implementation, raising the bar on their clinical education work and helping them solve problems that may have confounded and frustrated them. In this way, professional development can really serve to not only improve student outcomes but also improve job satisfaction for the clinical educator.

## Scholarship of Teaching and Learning Clinical Educator

It is at this level that clinical educators become researchers and engage with SoTL in order to investigate answers to their own unique questions. The clinical educator who cannot find a solution in the literature to a problem they are facing, the belief that they have found a unique

approach to clinical teaching and want to verify its effectiveness with data, and the clinical educator who adapts a method of clinical education that worked in a related field but hasn't been demonstrated in their own field—these are all opportunities where clinical educators may see the need to conduct clinical education research themselves. For reflective clinical educators who consider the whole of the EBE-CE model, they may see challenges that lie in the intersections between their responsibilities for patient outcomes, student outcomes, and their duties within the organization. In the development of the model, we see this as a mechanism for uncovering the "unconscious" aspects of clinical education that can better be explored in order to add more evidence to the pool of resources available (DeRuiter & Ginsberg, 2020; Ginsberg & DeRuiter, 2020). The SoTL clinical educator is ready to take the next step from reading and relying on evidence-based research to conducting their own research. We presume that if you are reading this book, you are either considering or have decided to take the step of moving to this level.

Being a SoTL clinical educator is the distinction between consuming evidence and producing your own. The process of producing your own is what the remainder of this workbook will help you with. We are here to walk you through many of the steps, including how to prepare to conduct the research, design it, collect the data, and disseminate the results. You don't need a research doctorate in order to be able to do this work! As a professional at this level, you are focusing much of your time and energy on the discovery of teaching and learning in the clinical setting, whether you are a part- or full-time clinical educator. The professional development you may look for at this stage may be content that will support your efforts, including organizations' presentations regarding clinical education approaches, as well as research methodologies. Consider that at the end of the process, by publishing and/or disseminating your work, you as the SoTL clinical educator are actually the one producing the knowledge that will in turn become professional development for other clinical educators.

# How to Find Research

One of the challenges of research, particularly if you are not employed by or currently enrolled as a student in a university, is gaining access to the literature and finding support for the search process. The challenge of figuring out how to access literature, even when it is available through your professional organization, has been shown to be significant (Davis et al., 2023). One of the ways to find your literature is to consider a variety of sources that you have available. You may find that some sources are easy to access and others can be challenging, but with persistence, you are likely to find just what you need.

# Sources

## Free and Open Access

There are a number of resources that are free and available to you, no matter your role, affiliation, or profession. Here are some examples:

- Directory of Open Access Journals (DOAJ; https://doaj.org): At the time of publication of this text, the DOAJ, which will help you find journals and journal articles that are completely free to all readers (hence *open access*), boasts inclusion of 19,671 journals and over 9 million articles. Please note that just because a journal is open access does not mean that it is a less quality journal. These journals are still peer-reviewed and should have the same level of rigorous review and publication process as journals that charge for subscriptions. Journals and articles represent a wide variety of disciplines and topics.

- Unpaywall (http://unpaywall.org): Unpaywall can help you find an article you are looking for by searching from an aggregate of sources, including the DOAJ and other open-access sources. This is an extension tool that you can add to Google Chrome to help you search for articles by DOI (digital object identifier) numbers. It is legal and is recommended by university librarians. There is no specific content focus for this service.

- Open Access Button (https://openaccessbutton.org): Open Access Button is similar to Unpaywall in that they do the search for you to obtain legal and free versions of full text articles from a large number of sources. If the item you are looking for cannot be found through their search, they have a requesting mechanism in which they will contact the author directly about making the article available to you free of charge. Similar to Unpaywall, they have browser extensions that can be added to your browser, or you can access them through their website.

- Education Resources Information Center (ERIC; https://eric.ed.gov): The focus of the ERIC database is content related to education (at all levels, including graduate and doctoral studies). You can search by limiting items to peer-reviewed resources or to those that are available as full texts free on ERIC. You are not guaranteed to find everything available as fully free text, as some content will lead to a pay/subscription portal, but much of it is and you may also find helpful reports that are not journal-specific. The Advanced Search Tips page is extremely helpful as well and will help you navigate the search process to find just the right items. More about finding those subscription limited items follows.

- MEDLINE/PubMed (https://pubmed.ncbi.nlm.nih.gov): MEDLINE and PubMed are the government-sponsored medicine and life science databases. They are funded by the National Library of Medicine in association with the National Institutes of Health. They offer free access to research that is generally health care–related. They can be a little trickier to navigate than some of the other databases, but they offer resources and user guides that will help you, particularly the MeSH system that uses specific vocabulary for searches.

- Google Scholar (https://scholar.google.com): Google Scholar will not guarantee you free and full access to all the literature that you find through a search, but it will give you information regarding what is available related to your topic. Some items, depending on where they were published and how old they are, may be available for free, but many will be behind pay or subscription walls. However, if you are just starting out and would like to know what exists related to your topic, it may be very helpful to you. At the very least, you will be able to read the article's abstract, which may help you determine if it is worth your time to continue to hunt down the article. One of the things that some researchers appreciate about Google Scholar that is unique is the ability to set up a profile that will notify you of new work by authors you are following or by topic words you are focused on. It will also offer you suggestions of work you may be interested in based on the profile you create.

## Affiliation-Based

You may learn, with a little digging, that you have access to a number of journals within your discipline through your professional organization. In our experience, many clinicians don't realize either how many resources professional organizations make available or how to navigate them. We recommend you explore the professional organizations or groups you are affiliated with to see what materials are available to you. You are probably already paying for a membership fee, so look into what access you have as part of that fee. Depending on the size of the organization you work for, you may also be able to access journal articles through your affiliation with your employer. Inquire as to whether or not they have any subscription services to peer-reviewed journals that you may be eligible to access.

If you cannot find a resource that you desperately want to get your hands on and it requires a subscription or a download fee, we would encourage you to think creatively about how you might access the article. You may find a former university mentor or the university internship coordinator you interact with would be willing to get the article for you. Additionally, a member of your board of mentors (see Chapter 5) might be able to serve as a resource. If you provide a mentor with the specific link to the article or the DOI number, this is a fairly simple task and is not a large favor. You may also find the paper's author contact information is visible on the page that hosts the abstract. It is worth emailing them (even if you have to Google them to figure out what their current email address is) and ask if they would be willing to provide you with a PDF of the article. You might be amazed at how many researchers are pleased to know that someone is interested in their work and more than happy to share with you.

## Search Strategies

There are many strategies people employ in order to find the articles that will be useful to them. Whichever strategy you use, you may find that it is helpful to take notes on your search process (Pittsley-Sousa, 2017). This will help you keep track of what you have done, what has worked, what hasn't worked, and ideas you have that you would like to explore as you move forward. For many of us, searching for literature can become a dive into a series of rabbit holes that you can get lost in. The notes you take will help keep you focused and organized. These notes might also be useful to you if you are engaging with a mentor who has specific questions about your approach.

In order to learn more about strategies you can use for literature searches, we will outline a few key steps and considerations here. However, know that if you look at many university library's websites (most of which are publicly available), they will also provide you with excellent resources and suggestions about how to be successful with this process.

### Key Words

Key words are the terms that you are probably thinking about in association with your topic. For example, if you are looking for information about clinical education in a hospital setting, you might search for the key words "clinical education" and "hospital." Databases typically let you look for more than one key word at a time, which will provide you with more focused information that is likely to be specific to your interests. However, if you narrow the search too much, you may discover that you don't find enough information. Therefore, sometimes it can be to your advantage when you are searching a new topic to search more broadly and scan some of the topics to get ideas of how you might want to narrow your search moving forward.

Remember that key words must be contained within the database in order for your search to yield maximum results. You may want to think of synonyms that might help you find more literature. For example, if you are looking for information about clinical education for clinicians working with children with a specific diagnosis, you might search for the diagnosis and "student clinician." However, depending on the database you are searching in, you may find additional materials if you search "intern," "resident," or "novice clinician." Know that different databases sometimes use different key words, so it is worth your time to think about the options or use a thesaurus. As you become more familiar with the literature on your topic, you may develop more specific key words or phrases, such as "self-efficacy" that will likely result in fewer items, but those that are listed may be particularly valuable to you.

### Boolean Operators

When you are searching a database that lets you enter more than one key word, you may see you are allowed to indicate the level of requirement or preference regarding that particular key word. The use of Boolean operators allows you to specify the combinations of terms that you are interested in (University of Leeds, n.d.). The most common Boolean operators are as follows:

- Or (used to find content that mentions either of the key words you entered)
- And (will find content that mentions both of the key words you entered)
- Not (will avoid key words you do not want to be included)

We recommend that you keep track of not only which key words you search for but also the Boolean operators that you use in your searches to avoid duplication of efforts and identify which approaches yield the best results for you.

## References and Citation Searches

Once you find a really relevant article that makes you feel like you struck gold, you can use it to find more. One way to do this is search through the reference list of that article and see what you find there that may have informed the work and could be valuable to you. Often the reference list of a research article will include work that is very similar to or has informed the work described in the article. If this article is particularly relevant but older, it may represent a good opportunity to learn more about the history of the topic and help you trace the evolution of thinking regarding it. This can be useful to you to understand as you move forward with your work.

Another strategy that may be helpful to you is to look for other work that has cited the article you have found to be valuable to you. How you do this will vary slightly depending on the database you are in. Using Google Scholar as an example, because it is always available to everyone, when you find the article you are hoping to find more similar ones to, click on "cited by" to find research that referenced that article or choose "related articles" to find more options the database thinks has commonalities with the one you are starting with.

## Think Broadly

Often when we begin a new search, we tend to think in fairly specific terms, including looking for research that is closest to home, so to speak. This may lead us to look for work that has been done on a topic from within our own discipline and perhaps from within our own context. While this is a terrific place to start, it isn't a great place to stop. Consider exploring related professions or related contexts. As a speech-language pathologist, I can tell you that I have learned about approaches to clinical education from medicine, psychology, and nursing that are useful. Branch out beyond your own discipline, particularly when you hit dead ends, to see what has been done by colleagues that might inform your thinking or practice. Similarly, while you find yourself working in a specific context and may be searching for research relevant to that context, consider if you broaden your search to include similar or related contexts. While you might not find that the concepts have 100% overlap and applicability to your interest, you may learn some new ideas that can be applied or modified for your setting.

## Types of Resources

### Research Journals

When you conduct your literature search using the strategies just described, you may find materials that represent peer-reviewed research, textbooks, and conference papers. Let's take a few minutes to identify what the differences are and how they might be useful to you. The first category is original research or primary literature. This is literature that reports results of research that the authors conducted. Primary research may be reporting on any type of study design (see Chapters 6 and 7). If you would like to learn about how the research was conducted, with which participants, and in what context, along with the specific outcome, then this article is going to be helpful to you to guide your EBP or to help you develop your research ideas.

If the research is published in an academic or professional journal, such as one oriented toward your discipline, it is likely to have been *peer-reviewed*. Peer-reviewed means that other researchers and experts in the field reviewed the study to determine that it met certain criteria, as specified by the journal. Peer-reviewed articles aren't guaranteed to be without flaws, but they should have passed through a rigorous review process prior to their publication.

There are several types of research papers that can appear in this category. While you may see an individual report of a single study, you may also see papers that are labeled as reviews (e.g., meta-analyses, systematic reviews, scoping reviews). In these papers, an author has undertaken to summarize and synthesize all the literature that is available on a particular topic. These papers are intended to give

you less detail about who did what compared to a research report, but they give you a systematic assessment or overview of the topic. If you are looking for insights regarding the current best practices or trends in an area of work, systematic reviews can be an excellent way to begin. If the review is published in a peer-reviewed journal, then you can be assured that it has undergone the same type of review the individual research paper has gone through.

### Non-Journal Sources

In addition to the journal articles described before, you may find resources during your search that are not from journals at all. These items may include conference presentations, papers that are based on conference presentations, and textbooks. These items may or may not be peer-reviewed, depending on the process that was used to move them forward. Many conference presentations at professional conferences, such as those sponsored by the discipline's governing or organizing body, are likely to be peer-reviewed. The level of rigor is likely to be slightly less than the journal review process, but that does not mean they are not valuable. You may find a presentation that was offered by the same author of one of your research papers. That is a great opportunity to see or hear how the researcher thinks about their work and explains it in their own words.

Finally, we would be remiss if we did not mention online resources. We are all inundated with digital information coming at us on a daily basis for most of us. You may find yourself following the social media related to your profession or your role within an organization that is insightful and helpful. Similarly, there are many blogs out there written by people who have done extensive research and work within a field. The information that you get from these resources may be helpful in shaping your thinking or even furthering your literature search strategies. However, depending on the source, take them with a grain of salt. If the person posting is someone you have never heard of, they may or may not be sharing information that is evidence-based. One way to increase the trustworthiness of online materials is to not only consider the name and reputation of the author, but also or has no affiliation with an organization you are familiar with. We recommend that you look for online information that is either associated with a professional organization (xxxx.org) that you are aware of or look for material that is affiliated with a university (xxxx.edu). Once you read these blogs, social media posts, and become familiar with the content, follow up with the original sources they are referring to so that you are making the most informed decisions about the content. Figure 4-3, reproduced from a clinical guide to reading research, gives you an idea about what types of research literature might be useful for you, depending upon the level of knowledge you have and are looking for.

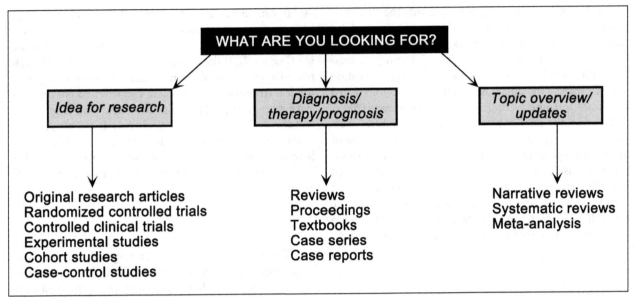

**Figure 4-3.** Schematic flow chart of the first step in choosing an article to read. (Reproduced with permission from Subramanyam, R. V. [2013]. Art of reading a journal article: Methodically and effectively. *Journal of Oral and Maxillofacial Pathology, 17*[1], 65-70. https://doi.org/10.4103/0973-029X.110733)

# READING RESEARCH

Learning how to quickly and efficiently read research to determine if it is of value to inform your EBP, whether clinical or educational, is critical to your success as a professional. It is not uncommon to hear that research is mystifying to read, and therefore, people might give up and avoid even trying to do so. If you are one of those folks, fear not—we are here to help! This section is designed to help you understand more about the anatomy of a research article, strategies for reading research, and how to evaluate if it might be useful in making decisions about your own work.

## Anatomy of a Research Article

What follows is a brief description of the content you can expect to find under each major heading of a research article. This may feel too rudimentary for some of you and that is okay. This information is provided for those who may be uncertain or uncomfortable with reading research so that we are all on the same page as we discuss strategies for reading research, which will come next. In addition to the brief overviews that will be shared here, you might also want to check the style guide (e.g., *Publication Manual of the American Psychological Association, Seventh Edition*) used for writing by your profession. You may see a little variability in formatting between articles written to conform to various style guidelines. However, the overall content should be consistent.

## Article Title

Aside from being the name of the article, it should give you a sense of what the article is about and the direction of the work. The title is what will probably either pique your interest or make you move on in search of other work. Be aware that titles don't always tell the full story regarding the focus of the article, so it is recommended that you think broadly about titles related to your search until you start narrowing down what will be most useful for you.

## Abstract

The abstract may be formatted by a variety of subheadings or by one brief paragraph. This varies mostly by journal preference. No matter how it is formatted, the abstract should tell you what the article is about: Is it a study, or is it a theoretical piece, or is it a reflection on EBP? It will tell you the most important elements of the paper. For a research article, it should include who was studied, what was the research question, what study methods were used, and key findings. The abstract is often what the reader will use to determine whether or not they want to keep reading the article.

## Introduction

The introduction should help explain the context of the work. It should explain to the reader why the topic is important and what we already know about it. The introduction will also review the relevant literature on the topic and then explain the current study differs from or adds to the work that has already been conducted. The introduction may also provide you with a *conceptual framework* for the study. A conceptual framework is a lens through which the researcher was looking through in collecting and analyzing the data. For example, a piece of clinical education research may be looking at how a clinical educator created significant learning according to Fink's taxonomy (2003). In that case, the introduction should include a brief overview of the Fink taxonomy (see Chapter 2 for a review of this taxonomy). Often the last item that appears in the introduction is the *research question* (sometimes abbreviated RQ). This is a specific and succinct statement as to what questions the researchers were trying to answer with the research. This will be an important part of your evaluation of the research as will be described in the following.

## Methods

The methods section of a research article will be broken down into several subheadings, such as research design, participants, data collection, and data analysis. This section will give you the details regarding what they did and how they did it. This information lets you make comparisons between the study and your own application of the research. Given that you may be trying to find research that helps you provide clinical or educational support in a particular setting, this section will help you figure out if the setting in which the study took place is comparable to your context, for example. Even if the settings differ somewhat, the study might yield valuable insights for you. It's just important to recognize the differences between the study's setting and your own so that you can adapt and account for it. This is also the section that will help you understand the methods used for analyzing the data you will read about in the next section. For many readers, we hear this is the most mystifying section, particularly when it comes to statistics. However, you can likely sort out much of what you need to know about the statistics with knowledge of a few key elements from Chapter 6. Unless you are trying to replicate the study you are reading about, the main focus in reading the methods section should be understanding what they did and how they did it. You should also ask yourself if you feel that the data they collected and analyzed, along with their other method details, seem appropriate to answering the research question (Subramanyam, 2013). If there seems to be a mismatch between the research question and the data that were collected, or who participated in the study, that might lead you to question the results and their inherent value to you.

## Results

In the results section, you will find out what the researchers learned. If they collected qualitative data through interviews, here you will learn about what the participants said during those interviews. You will also read here about how the researchers organized the results of the interviews in a meaningful way (coding and thematic analysis, see Chapter 7). If they collected quantitative data through objective measures of learning, such as memorizing anatomical structures, here is where you will find out how the learners performed based on how they were taught. You will also read about the statistical analysis and significance or interpretation of those findings. You may also learn more here about time frames for implementation, variability that occurred in the data, or additional information that is relevant to interpreting the data.

## Discussion

The discussion section, which might also include sections labeled *conclusions*, *limitations*, and *future directions*, is where the researchers delve into not only what they found but what it means and why it is important to us. Here they will connect the findings that were summarized in the literature review to the findings from the data and perhaps note that they agreed, disagreed, differed for some reason, or augmented what we previously knew about the topic. In this section the authors will also use the data that they reported in the results section to support conclusions they have come to and should be used to answer their research question(s). In addition to the conclusions regarding what was learned from this study, you are likely to find a few comments about the *limitations* of the study. This information is an acknowledgment by the authors of factors they were unable to control or account for, such as funding and time limitations, that may have influenced the outcome of their study. These recognitions should not necessarily be seen as shortcomings or failures on the part of the research, but more as transparency about the realities of research implementation.

## References and Appendices

At the very end of the article, you will find a reference list and possibly appendices. The reference list should include the full information regarding each and every source of information that appeared in the article you just read. The article's information is intended to be complete enough that you should be able to use it to find the article for yourself. This is important because as you are seeking out information that will be used to support your own EBPs, you might want information that provides further data, relevant background information, or even different, conflicting findings that the authors acknowledge in their writing. The reference list will help you find the sources. Following the references, you may find appendices. Not all articles will have these; however, if the authors want to share materials or information with you, such as the survey tool they used, the materials used for teaching, or the interview questions

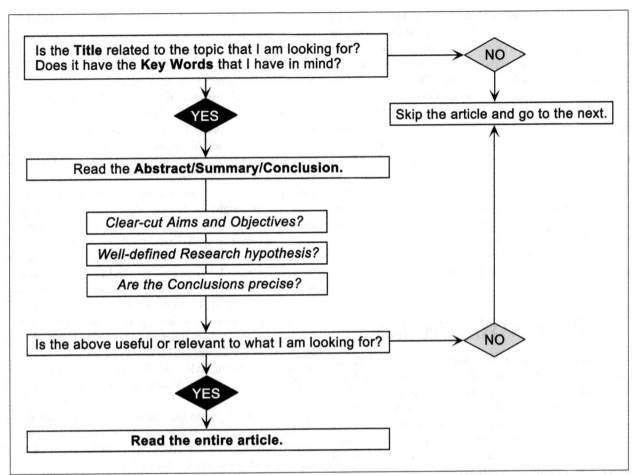

**Figure 4-4.** Decision-making flow chart to decide whether to read the chosen article or not. (Reproduced with permission from Subramanyam, R. V. [2013]. Art of reading a journal article: Methodically and effectively. *Journal of Oral and Maxillofacial Pathology, 17*[1], 65-70. https://doi.org/10.4103/0973-029X.110733)

that were asked, they will likely be included here. The inclusion of these materials can help you avoid reinventing the wheel or searching for it elsewhere.

# Reading Strategies

Reading the research can be a little tricky in that how you read it will depend in large part on why you are reading it in the first place. While it might seem obvious that you read a research article from the beginning straight through to the end, in the order that it was written, this actually is often not the case (Pain, 2016; Subramanyam, 2013; University of Minnesota Libraries, n.d.). The University of Minnesota Libraries (n.d.) video suggests that the best way to read an article is by using the ADIRM order: abstract, discussion, introduction, results, and then methods. Their rationale for this is that it's the most efficient way to determine if it's worth continuing to read or not. By reading the abstract first, you can decide if the article is going to be valuable to you for your purpose. Jumping to the discussion

allows you to discern if their results were relevant and valuable to the question at hand, while reading the introduction will tell you more about the background and the specifics of the research question. Reading the results will tell you what the actual data reflected. It is recommended to read the methods last because it is often overwhelming for people, but as noted before, if you read it carefully, you will be able to learn more about what was really done in the study and identify what aspects of it are least or most relevant to you.

A similar approach is advocated by Subramanyam (2013). Depicted as a flow chart in Figure 4-4, this model suggests that reading the title and key words first will help you decide if it's worth your time to continue reading at each step, beginning with the abstract and key words before going on to the summary and then conclusions.

Where I (SMG) start reading research articles depends on why I'm reading and what stage of the search I'm in. If I'm new to a topic and just trying to learn something about it, I'm likely to start with the introduction because I want to find out what researchers who are knowledgeable about the topic think is important and relevant background information that I need to understand. If I'm reading to find out if their approach to clinical education worked in the context of the study, I'll read the discussion first to see if what they learned was valuable to them and might also be valuable to me. In each of these cases, I'll make a decision as I read as to whether or not to continue reading. I don't finish each article, as this would not be an effective use of my time if I determine that what is written is not helpful or not applicable to me. Mark always makes sure to scan the reference list of articles, even when they don't "fit" the work you are trying to accomplish. Sometimes there can be a gem you might have missed that informs your future searches. While there are a number of different ways to approach reading research articles, the thing we want you to know is that reading from start to finish is seldom in your best interest. As you read more research, you will develop your own patterns that work for you.

## Organizing What You Read

As you move through this chapter and consider all that there is to find in the literature and all that you have to learn from each article, you might start to feel overwhelmed by how much there is to read and keep track of. You might be wondering how best to manage the mountain of information you are about to climb. The honest answer is that there is absolutely no one right way to do it. It is an individualized process, led by individual preferences.

Here are a few of the ways that colleagues manage the process. If you are a technology person and prefer apps and programs to make your life simple, you might look at one of the many online resources that are available for tracking and organizing references. For example, Carol C. Dudding, Chapter 3's author, likes Zotero (www.zotero.org) for managing references and sharing resources. She notes: There are a number of low-cost/no-cost citation managers available for your use (e.g., Zotero, Endnote, Mendeley). Most systems will allow you to upload the articles and/or the URL making it easy to retrieve later on. When selecting a citation manager, you may want to choose one that is web-based so that you can add to and access the information from any device or browser. Zotero makes adding an article to your collection as easy as clicking on a plug-in that is added to your browser. This works much like Pinterest. Whatever citation manager you decide to go with, it is definitely worth the time and effort to set up and use a citation manager. There are online tools that organizations may subscribe to, such as RefWorks (www.refworks.com), that are not free, but affiliation with one of your organizations may gain you access. Additionally, you might want to check to see if your professional organization or your employer might have access to one of these tools.

Chapter 8 co-author Jordan Dann likes using technology but doesn't use one of the online webtools. Jordan uses a combination of creating Excel spreadsheets and multiple folders on his hard drive to sort and track the articles that he finds in the search process. This is a process that works well for him and helps him feel organized as he collects articles and prepares to write. And then there is me (SMG). I'm old-school. I prefer to print out all the articles that I want to read and will likely use for my work. I then annotate them right on the paper, using a combination of regular pens, highlighters, and sometimes the tiny sticky notes that you can use to flag single lines of text (similar to the tiny ones that you might see that say "sign here"). I then write a few key words on the top right corner of the article to annotate it and remind myself what is particularly important (or sometimes I note that the article wasn't at all useful to me). Similar to Jordan, I organize my articles in folders, but mine are regular file folders, not digital ones, so that I can find the materials I need at a later date. My only concession to technology at this stage of reading the literature is to create what I label as a "Master Reference Sheet" for each study or topic. In a Word document, I create a reference list, formatted according to the style guide for my profession, that has all the references I have read included. That way I don't have to stop and check to see if I have added the reference for anything that I might do later, such as write a research article. Mark notes that he is somewhere in between paper and technology, downloading articles to his tablet and marking them up with the electronic tablet pencil.

Another old-school approach that you may have been asked to do as a student is to create an annotated bibliography. Some of the online tools will help you do this, or you can essentially do it in a digital spreadsheet or on paper. I teach graduate students to write an annotated bibliography when they begin searching for literature in graduate school. I'm not fussy about the format they use or how it is organized. I want them to develop a process that works for them. But I do suggest there are some key elements that should be included because I think it will make the research process easier for them. An annotated bibliography can also be helpful if you are collaborating with colleagues because it can help you share what you have learned with them and also keep you from duplicating each other's work. Here are some of my suggestions for what to include in your annotated bibliography:

- Reference: List the article in the reference list format dictated by your style guide.

- Summary: Write a sentence or two of what the article is about or what research found.

- Assess: Compare it to other articles, describe if it feels useful or informative or unhelpful.

- Reflect: Consider how this article relates to your work. Is a specific aspect useful?

The bottom line is that whatever process works for you is absolutely the best. Just like finding your way to writing good clinical documentation, there is no one size fits all in figuring out how to get there. You just need to be sure that you are organized so that you make good use of your time and are able to find what you need at a later date should the need arise. A final thing to consider is your time. Sometimes learning an entirely new system can be a time saver. In other instances, it is a time waster because you are not dealing with a volume of information that is great enough to make the new process worth it in the long-term.

# Evaluating Research

As you read through the research that you have found, it can be difficult to critically appraise the quality of the information. We often hear that people are intimidated by reading research. That may have something to do with feeling like you don't have enough knowledge about the research process to assess whether the information is good or not. However, with a little guidance, we think that you can confidently assess the quality of the literature you are reading. The most important thing to remember is that while the peer review process is there to improve the quality of what is published, it is not 100% foolproof. It is possible to see articles published that have slipped through cracks of peer checking and sometimes are even retracted by the journal when they discover an inconsistency or falsification in the research. So while the vast majority of work out there can be trusted, we recommend that you assess it yourself.

# Assessing Integrity and Trustworthiness

Your first read of an article should give you an overall sense of how clear the paper is. Ask yourself if the terminology is well defined, if the research question is explained clearly. When you look at the people who were studied, was the sample representative of a subset of individuals (e.g., all men) or of all people who might be studied. There might be a good reason to study a subset of individuals within a potentially larger group, such as that is who the researcher was interested in learning about, but do the conclusions speak to the people in the study or to a wider group of individuals than were studied? Does the study's design make sense as it is described, and does it appear designed to answer the research question posed by the authors? When you read the discussion and conclusion sections, does the interpretation of the results make sense in the context of the study? Do the authors appropriately acknowledge the limitations of the study and how the data may be useful? As you read

through the article, there should be a flow that allows you to make connections between each of the elements described such that each seems logical to you. A study that was done well but was poorly written may not be valuable to you. Finally, as you are probably reading an individual study in the context of several other studies on the same topic, ask yourself how the article fits in with what you have already read. Does there appear to be general agreement across the studies, and do they fit in well together, expanding knowledge rather than contradicting it?

# Assessing Statistics

We are going to address the one thing that we suspect is often the source of preventing readers from trying to consume or use research more: statistics. While Chapter 6 will address several specific types of research statistics, we are going to focus on how to interpret the results or the *p* value, or probability. Unless you are an avid researcher and an expert in statistical analysis, you are likely to not recognize the names of all the statistical tests that could be conducted in quantitative research. That is okay—don't stop reading! What is perhaps most critical to understand about almost all statistical analyses is that they are mathematical calculations designed to determine if the outcomes in the study were random chance or if they were a reflection of the study's intervention. This concept is termed *statistical significance*. Findings of statistical significance suggest to the reader that the outcome of the study was due to whatever manipulations or interventions the researchers conducted during the study. Think of probability as ranging from 0 to 1. If the probability that the relationship between the variable study and the outcome is 0, that means there is no chance it was related. The outcome would have occurred no matter what the researchers did. On the other hand, if the probability is 1, then it is absolutely certain that there is a relationship between what the researchers did and the outcome of the study. In quantitative research, we never make an assumption of guaranteed, perfect certainty of the results. Therefore, if you think about the results with a probability of nearly 1 or .99, then that suggests a *p* value of .01 where the *p* value represents the slimmest chance that the outcome was unrelated to study. This is the lowest *p* value we will see reported and is the strongest outcome we can expect. A *p* value of .05 means that the researchers are 95% sure the outcome wasn't by chance and was related to their interventions. This is considered the minimum level for indicating statistical significance. A *p* value higher than .05 suggests that the researchers could not be at least 95% confident they influenced the outcome of the study, and therefore, no clear conclusions can be drawn. Keep in mind this doesn't mean that there was no relationship between the intervention and the outcome, but it means that we cannot say there was with any certainty. As you read statistical analyses, remember that you are looking for the smallest possible *p* value, between .01 and .05, to indicate the outcomes of the study were significant.

## ASSESSING GENERALIZABILITY

Finally, we would like to conclude with a word about generalizability of the research you read. Generalizability means that you are able to take the results of a study based on a sample population and apply it to a larger population or the whole population. It implies the transferability of the results to everyone who shares the characteristics of the individuals being studied. Quantitative research, particularly studies that have very large groups of participants (often referred to as having a large *N* where *N* = number of participants) derive much of their power from the fact that they are more likely to represent wide swaths of the population being studied. For example, if you consider standardized assessments, such as IQ tests, many hundreds of thousands of people have taken these tests, increasing the likelihood that no matter your age or gender, the results can reasonably be assumed to represent you. As such, the results are said to be *generalizable* to the wider population. Clinical and educational studies often have much smaller groups (small *n*), but still have enough participants to be able to conduct statistical analyses and suggest that the results apply to a wide range of individuals within the population of people being studied.

One of the criticisms of case studies, single-subject studies, and qualitative studies is that they lack generalizability. In the purest statistical sense of the term, this is true in that the results from a small number of people cannot be presumed to represent a large percentage of the population (specifically and more accurately referred to as statistical-probabilistic generalizability). And while most journals will essentially expect a study with a small number of participants, including qualitative research (see Chapter 7) to note that the results are not generalizable, this undermines the value of these studies. The primary issue is many readers assume that a study whose results are not generalizable is not valuable, it can be disregarded as not being useful to guide EBP or EBE. For quantitative research, generalizability is a standard and an implied positive characteristic, while for qualitative work and studies with small participant pools, it is typically noted as a shortcoming. It suggests that the research offers little to be learned and applied to the reader's context because it wasn't big enough. This isn't true and suggests a bias toward quantitative studies.

If, on the other hand, we consider that there is more than one type of generalizability, beyond the statistical one, then we might be able to appreciate the value inherent in the small participant research studies. Two additional types of generalizability should be considered in the context of these studies and how useful they are at informing our work (Smith, 2018):

1. Naturalistic generalizability: The research resonates with the reader's experiences.
2. Transferability or inferential generalizability: The extent to which the outcomes from the study can be applied to the context in which the reader is working.

In other words, the measure that should be applied to case studies and qualitative research should not be the same as the standard used in quantitative research. Rather, it is critical that as you read the work, you reflect on if the information feels credible and authentic (Creswell, 2003; Denzin & Lincoln, 2003) and learning from the studies can be applied to the context in which you are practicing.

## SUMMING IT UP

This chapter has given you many great things to consider. Some of the concepts will be reinforced in other chapters (e.g., quantitative and qualitative research) and other concepts will be ones you'll be able to put into practice as you begin to conduct your own work. The main point is this: Asking research questions starts a cycle of inquiry. Sometimes the information you find will be clear and helpful to the questions you are asking. Other information might be challenging or contradict your original thoughts and questions. The main point here is to start your journey into evidence with an open mind and push yourself to search and read beyond your boundaries!

# REFERENCES

Creswell, J. W. (2003). *Research design: Qualitative, quantitative, and mixed methods approaches* (2nd ed.). Sage.

Davis, R. A., Brundage, S. B., Garber, M., Bocchino, J. M., & Ginsberg, S. M. (2023). *Speech-language pathologists' perspectives on evidence-based practice in the healthcare setting: A qualitative study.* [Doctor of Philosophy in Translational Health Sciences Dissertations. Paper 20. George Washington University.] https://hsrc.himmelfarb.gwu.edu/smhs_crl_dissertations/20

Denzin, N. K., & Lincoln, Y. S. (2003). Introduction: The discipline and practice of qualitative research. In N. K. Denzin & Y. S. Lincoln (Eds.), *Strategies of qualitative inquiry* (2nd ed., pp. 1-45). Sage.

DeRuiter, M., & Ginsberg, S. M. (2020). Conscious clinical education: The evidence-based education-clinical education model. *Seminars in Speech and Language, 41*(4), 279-288. https://doi.org/10.1055/s-0040-1713779

Filipe, H. P., Silva, E. D., Stulting, A. A., & Golnik, K. C. (2014). Continuing professional development: Best practices. *Middle East African Journal of Ophthalmology, 21*(2), 134-141.

Fink, L. D. (2003). *Creating significant learning experiences: An integrated approach to designing college courses.* Jossey-Bass.

Ginsberg, S. M., & DeRuiter, M. (2020). Research and the clinical education and supervision process. In E. S. McCrea & J. A. Brasseur (Eds.), *The clinical education and supervisory process in speech-language pathology and audiology.* SLACK Incorporated.

Institute of Medicine. (2010). *Redesigning continuing education in the health professions.* The National Academies Press. https://www.ncbi.nlm.nih.gov/books/NBK219811/

McKinney, K. (2007). *Enhancing learning through the scholarship of teaching and learning: The challenges and joys of juggling.* Anker.

Pain, E. (2016, March). How to (seriously) read a scientific paper. *Science.* https://www.science.org/content/article/how-seriously-read-scientific-paper

Pittsley-Sousa, K. (2017). *Finding the right words.* Eastern Michigan University. https://guides.emich.edu/csd/tutorials

Roberts, D. H., Schwartzstein, R. M., & Weinberger, S. E. (2014). Career development for the clinician-educator. *Annals American Thoracic Society, 11*(2), 254-259. https://doi.org/10.1513/AnnalsATS.201309-322OT

Smith, B. (2018). Generalizability in qualitative research: misunderstandings, opportunities and recommendations for the sport and exercise sciences. *Qualitative Research in Sport, Exercise and Health, 10*(1), 137-149. https://doi.org/10.1080/2159676X.2017.1393221

Stein, A. M. (2021). History of continuing nursing education in the United States. *Journal of Continuing Education in Nursing, 29*(6), 245-252. https://doi.org/10.3928/0022-0124-19981101-04

Subramanyam, R. V. (2013). Art of reading a journal article: Methodically and effectively. *Journal of Oral and Maxillofacial Pathology, 17*(1), 65-70. https://www.ncbi.nlm.nih.gov/pmc/articles/PMC3687192/

Traylor, K. M., Cervantes, J. L., & Perry, C. N. (2020). Professional development track to prepare future academic clinicians. *Medical Science Educator, 31*, 24-27.

University of Leeds. (n.d.). *Literature searching explained.* https://library.leeds.ac.uk/info/1404/literature_searching/14/literature_searching_explained/4#search%20terms

University of Minnesota Libraries. (n.d.). *How to read and comprehend scientific research articles* [Video]. https://www.youtube.com/watch?v=t2K6mJkSW0A

# Worksheet 4-1:
# Research as Professional Development

What are your professional roles (refer to Chapter 1 for review of roles), and what are your learning needs for each?

| Roles | Learning Needs |
|---|---|
|  |  |
|  |  |
|  |  |
|  |  |
|  |  |

## Identifying Professional Development Needs and Opportunities in Clinical Education

For the learning needs identified above, consider your professional development level for learning about the topic. You may be a different level for different topics.

1. Look for the literature on the topic. (Good clinical educator)
2. Read the literature on the topic. (Scholarly clinical educator)
3. Ready to investigate the topic yourself. (SoTL clinical educator)

| Clinical Education Questions/Challenges/Opportunities | Professional Development Level (Good, Scholarly, SoTL) |
|---|---|
|  |  |
|  |  |
|  |  |
|  |  |
|  |  |

# A Board of Mentors to Support Clinical Education Research

*Lizbeth H. Finestack, PhD, CCC-SLP*

As a clinical educator, you likely have many areas of expertise that will assist you as you embark on conducting clinical education research. For example, you likely have expertise in providing high-quality, evidence-based services to clients. It is also likely that you have developed effective methods to help students grow their own clinical skills. Your expertise in clinical practice and education provides you with the essential foundation needed as you begin to evaluate methods and approaches surrounding clinical education. If you reflect on your training that has allowed you to get to this point in your professional career, it is also likely that you received much support along the way from people, such as instructors, supervisors, peers, and even your clients and students. As you work to expand your professional skills and gain expertise in conducting clinical education research, it is no different. You will need support and guidance from many individuals to help to ensure your success. You need *mentorship*. I purposefully use the term mentorship here to help convey that the guidance and support you need is multifaceted. There will likely be several individuals who you will need to help guide you as you gain skills in several different areas over time. Thus, one model that may serve you well for clinical education research, given its complexities, is a board of mentors.

## What Is a Board of Mentors?

As you will see in each of the chapters that follow, there are many aspects of clinical education research for you to consider, including conducting a review of research related to your area of interest (Chapter 4); developing your research question(s) (Chapters 4 and 8); determining the study design (Chapter 8); developing the study protocol (Chapter 9); gaining approval to conduct research (Chapter 9); recruiting and consenting participants (Chapter 9); collecting, processing, and analyzing data (Chapters 6 and 7); and disseminating your findings through presentations and/or manuscripts (Chapters 11 and 12). Likewise, there are a variety of areas for which you should consider seeking mentorship to support you. As you identify these areas, you will need to determine *who* can provide you support. It would be a very rare occurrence for the *who* to be a single person. It is unlikely that a single person will have the necessary expertise for each area of needed support. Moreover, in the unlikely event that they did, it would be doubtful that

DeRuiter, M., & Ginsberg, S. M. (Eds.). *Clinician's Guide to Applying, Conducting, and Disseminating Clinical Education Research* (pp. 49-58).
© 2024 Taylor & Francis Group.

they have the necessary time to support you, as these individuals are probably professionals with careers of their own to maintain. Thus, you should consider building a board of mentors to support your clinical education research.

You might be saying to yourself, "What is a 'board of mentors?' That sounds serious." A board of mentors is simply a composition of people that you assemble to support you. This is similar to a board of directors that a Fortune 500 company may have that comprises individuals such as the chief executive officer, the chief financial officer, shareholders, and employees. Each board member has different areas of expertise, but they all work together to make decisions to ensure the success of the business. Similarly, you can think of your board of mentors as individuals with different areas of expertise who have the collective goal of your success in clinical education research. Unlike a board of directors, it is not the intent that your board of mentors will all come together simultaneously to discuss your project. You may meet with some in small groups, but it is more likely that you will meet with your mentors individually.

# WHO ARE MY BOARD OF MENTORS?

Your next question is probably, "Who should comprise my 'board of mentors?'" You will need to find at least one person with expertise in each given area who is willing and has the time to support you. It is likely that one person can help support a few areas. It may also be useful to have multiple people within a single area who you identify as mentors. Table 5-1 provides a list of some potential mentors along with potential areas for which they can provide support.

Let's consider an example to demonstrate how you may utilize expertise from several individuals with different areas of knowledge. For this example, your board of mentors will comprise some of the individuals listed in Table 5-1. In practice, your board of mentors may include fewer or more individuals, with the same or different areas of expertise. Your board of mentors will need to be individualized to your unique research questions and needs.

## Example

### Background

Imagine that you have been providing clinical supervision for several *students*. Because of scheduling conflicts, you meet with some students individually weekly and others in a small group weekly. In passing conversation, one of the students in the small group alluded that they wished

they could meet with you individually to get more support. You quickly responded, "If only there was more time in a day!" Upon considering this comment and reflecting on the progress made by the students you meet with individually compared to those you meet in small groups, your impression is that students who meet in small groups demonstrate greater clinical gains. You hypothesize that this is likely because a student meeting in a small group may begin implementing feedback provided to other students before the individual student receives the feedback themselves. This prompts you to go through the following steps.

### Step 1

You decide to better understand differences between individual and group supervision meetings. You reach out to two students, one with whom you have been meeting with in a small group and another with whom your supervisor has been meeting with individually. You schedule a 30-minute meeting with the two of them together. At the beginning of the meeting, you explain that the purpose of the meeting is to help you to develop a list of pros and cons for individual and group meetings. You stress that you highly value each of their input and they should feel comfortable being honest and open. You explain that their comments and feedback will not affect their relationship with you, and if at any time they feel uncomfortable or have concerns, they should consult your supervisor. Through the meeting, you gain the students' perspectives of potential advantages and disadvantages of each supervisory model, with no model having a clear advantage over the other.

### Step 2

Given the feedback you received from the students, you are unsure if your impression that students who you meet in small groups make greater gains in their clinical skills than students who meet individually, but you would like to know the answer to this question to guide your supervision and scheduling of students in the future. You decide to meet with a *colleague* with whom you work closely, as well as your *supervisor* to see what thoughts they have on this topic and if they have had similar experiences. Your colleague asserts that they always meet with their students in small groups, while your supervisor reports only meeting with students individually. They both express that this is an interesting question they would like to know the answer to as well.

### Step 3

Given your colleagues' shared interest in this question, you decide to pursue the topic further. You develop a PICO (population/problem, intervention, comparator/control,

| | |
|---|---|
| **Table 5-1** | |

### POTENTIAL MENTORS AND CORRESPONDING AREAS OF SUPPORT

| POTENTIAL MENTOR | POTENTIAL AREA(S) OF SUPPORT |
|---|---|
| Student | • Providing feedback regarding clinical education experiences<br>• Identifying research topic<br>• Researching current evidence base<br>• Developing study protocol<br>• Collecting and processing data |
| Colleague | • Identifying research topic<br>• Developing research questions<br>• Developing study protocol<br>• Collecting and processing data<br>• Presenting study and results |
| Supervisor | • Identifying research topic<br>• Developing research questions<br>• Developing study protocol<br>• Gaining research approval<br>• Collecting and processing data<br>• Presenting study and results |
| Client | • Identifying research topic<br>• Developing study protocol |
| Community member | • Identifying research topic |
| Professor/instructor/researcher | • Researching current evidence base<br>• Developing research questions<br>• Determining study design<br>• Gaining research approval<br>• Analyzing data<br>• Presenting study and results<br>• Publishing study results |
| Graduate/PhD student | • Researching current evidence base<br>• Developing research questions<br>• Determining study design<br>• Gaining research approval<br>• Collecting and processing data<br>• Analyzing data<br>• Presenting study and results<br>• Publishing study results |
| Statistician | • Determining study design<br>• Analyzing data<br>• Publishing study results |

and outcome) question, as described in Chapter 1, but you wonder if the answer to this question has already been determined. You know that you need to examine the existing evidence base for individual vs. group supervisory models. Using strategies presented in Chapter 3, you complete a brief review of existing research, but you feel unsure of your approach. You decide to reach out to a *professor* that you had in graduate school for help. The instructor is interested in your project and provides you with additional resources for conducting your research review.

## Step 4

After spending time reviewing the literature base, you find that there is limited evidence available to address your PICO question. You share the results of your literature review with your *supervisor* and *colleague*. They remain excited about your PICO question and encourage you to conduct your own evaluation of supervisory models.

## Step 5

You go back to your former *professor* to talk about the possibility of conducting your own study. The professor agrees that it is a worthwhile project and believes that you could conduct your own investigation with support. The professor explains that you will need to complete trainings for working with human participants and provides you with training resources offered through the professor's institution.

## Step 6

Once you complete the necessary training, you meet with the professor to talk about potential study designs you could use. The professor suggests that you consult their advanced *PhD student* who has recently completed a series of research methods and analyses courses. The three of you meet to design the study.

## Step 7

After designing your study, you meet with your *colleague* and *supervisor* again to discuss details about your protocol, study implementation, and the data you will be collecting. You also meet with the two *students* you met with in Step 1 to ask for their input regarding the project protocol. They are eager to serve as student mentors for your project.

## Step 8

Once you have determined your study protocol, you go back to your former professor to ask about the next steps. The professor reminds you that you will need to acquire institutional review board (IRB) approval for the protection of human participants for your study before you can consent student participants and begin collecting data (see Chapter 9 for more about IRB). The professor shares with you an IRB application they used for a previous study and encourages you to meet with the *PhD student* with questions regarding the application.

## Step 9

Upon gaining IRB approval, you begin conducting your study. You go to the *student* mentors and your *supervisor* for input on recruitment approaches and data collection logistics. You check in with the *professor* and *PhD student* on your progress.

## Step 10

Upon completing your data collection, you meet with the *PhD student* to discuss analyses and interpretation of your study results. You work with both the *PhD student* and the *professor* to disseminate your study findings through conference presentations and to submit a report to be considered for publication.

This simplified example serves to exemplify how a board of mentors can allow you to leverage the expertise of many different individuals as you conduct clinical education research, which is inherently complex and involves many steps. Figure 5-1 illustrates the mentors and some of their key roles in this example. The Board of Mentors Worksheet at the end of this chapter provides resources for you to use as you build your board of mentors.

# How Do I Find a Board of Mentors?

Before recruiting individuals to serve on your mentor board, it is important that you assess your needs and predict the areas for which you need mentorship support. Each chapter of this text provides valuable information regarding key components of clinical education research. Thus, as you read through each chapter, I encourage you to take notes of the research components and start thinking about individuals who could potentially mentor you in that area. The Board of Mentors Worksheet includes a blank mentoring planning table you may use as you design your board of mentors.

A natural beginning point to finding mentors for your board is to ask those around you. You can consider current students and peers, former colleagues, and former instructors, among others. As you talk to them about your research ideas, they may refer you to others to contact. A referral source will help provide a context to individuals you contact who you do not know. You may also search for mentors at local colleges and universities. You can start by using the internet to find professors, instructors, and/or students with similar areas of interest, then introducing yourself via email, and asking if they would have time for a short in-person meeting or tele-meeting. Professional conferences and conventions are also good venues for increasing your professional network. You may attend sessions on relevant topics, then speak to presenters at the conference or through follow-up communication

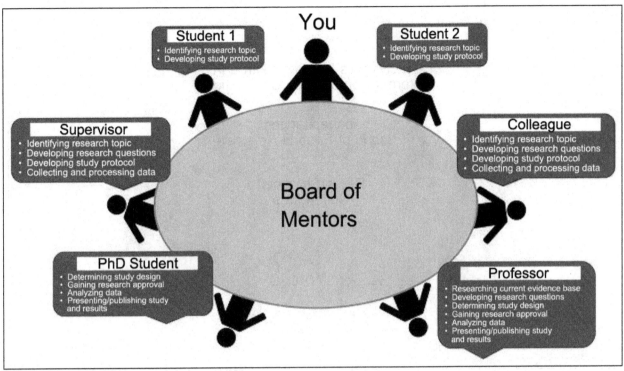

**Figure 5-1.** Example board of mentors with example roles.

after the conference. Your professional organization may also be a source for identifying potential mentors. For example, the American Speech-Language-Hearing Association has an online community, Clinicians & Researchers Collaborating (American Speech-Language-Hearing Association, n.d.), designed for researchers and clinicians to discuss and share ideas, advice, and resources on research collaborations. The American Physical Therapy Association Academy of Research has an Evidence-Based Practice Special Interest Group designed to provide a "forum for clinicians, educators and researchers that promotes collaboration and innovation for informed application of research evidence in practice" (n.d.). The American Academy of Physician Associates (n.d.) offers fellowships, as well as research events and "huddles," that allow for collaborative opportunities. Figure 5-2 illustrates differing relationship proximities for you to consider when building your board of mentors.

As you are identifying individuals to be a part of your board, there are multiple factors for you to consider. You will want to ensure that the mentor's area of expertise matches your needs. In addition to an area of expertise, you will want to ensure that the mentor will serve a supportive role. Following are descriptions of characteristics (Nakamura & Shernoff, 2009) that you should consider when choosing a mentor:

- *Supportive:* Mentors should be supportive of your desire to conduct clinical education research and also supportive of your specific research ideas and approaches. This does not mean that mentors should always agree with your viewpoints. Instead, the mentor should offer a critical eye to support the success of the project.

- *Involved:* Each mentor will have a different level of involvement; however, it is essential that if an individual is identified as a mentor, they be involved to some degree. Some mentors may only be involved in one or two short-term components of the research project, while others may be involved in all components for the entire project duration.

- *Balance freedom and guidance:* While each mentor may possess expertise in many areas applicable to your project, it is always important to remember that it is ultimately your project. The mentor should offer you guidance and suggestions, but the final decisions will be yours. Thus, it will be important to identify mentors that respect and allow for your freedom in project decision making.

- *Provide resources:* In addition to providing comments, suggestions, and feedback regarding your project, a mentor should also provide resources that will allow you to build your own knowledge base and expertise. Such resources may include pertinent published studies, books related to the research content, and books that support the research process. Resources may also include introductions to individuals with other areas of expertise to increase your network and information about conferences and conventions that may support your research. Other resources that a mentor may be able to provide include access to participants, IRB, libraries, and research assistants.

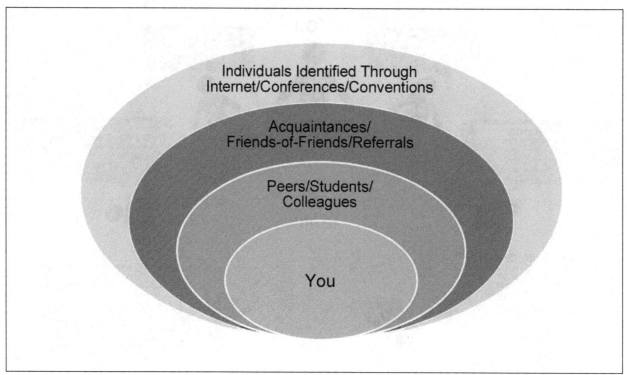

**Figure 5-2.** Proximal relationships of sources to consider when identifying mentors.

- *Provide frequent, positive feedback:* Frequent communication with a mentor will ensure that the mentor stays informed of the project progress. It will allow you to discuss decisions as you are making them instead of after the fact, when it may be too late to make changes. Additionally, while you want a mentor to offer critical and thoughtful comments and feedback, it is important the mentor is able to provide suggestions that will build and improve the project. It is also helpful for a mentor to provide positive reinforcement to highlight your growth and achievements and to help you build confidence and motivation to complete the project.

- *Treat you as a respected collaborator:* Although in many cases a mentor may be accustomed to approaching mentoring from a place of authority and power, mentorship works best when both the mentee and mentor are treated as respected equals. The mentor-mentee relationship is a collaborative relationship with both parties sharing the same goals: project success. As you identify mentors, make certain that they will come to the relationship as an excited collaborator who is eager to work *with* you.

Along with these positive characteristics to seek in a mentor, there are characteristics and behaviors that you will want to avoid, such as abuse, extreme self-interest, and neglect. A mentor should not exhibit any behaviors that are abusive, offensive, or hostile, such as behaviors that are intimidating, threatening, humiliating; behaviors that use

condescending, humiliating, or vulgar language, swearing, or shouting; and comments and behaviors that are sexist, racist, homophobic, xenophobic, or otherwise offensive (Disrupting Academic Bullying, n.d.). An individual who is abusive in any way or who bullies should not be considered a mentor.

### Box 5-1:
### Academic Bullying

Bullying can occur in any work environment, and academia is not immune to this situation. Gewin (2021) discusses bullying in an academic setting and ways to mitigate it. Remember that the first step will be to recognize the bullying behavior. Negative comments that are professionally and appropriately delivered are *not* bullying. However, extreme responses to situations that might be considered "small" could be considered inappropriate. Additionally, ridiculing, blaming, or any kind of threat could be considered bullying behavior. If you feel you are being bullied, Gewin recommends seeking support, exploring any routes you might have for a complaint, and fully understanding what the follow-through will be should you register a complaint.

Because a mentor's role is to support you, a mentor should not allow their self-interests to interfere with the support they offer you. An individual that exhibits comments or behaviors that ignore your concerns and contributions or that fails to give you appropriate credit for your work is not a valuable mentor. Additionally, you want to ensure that a mentor provides you with the appropriate support in terms of time and resources and that you and your project are not neglected. The amount of support a mentor provides will vary greatly, most important is that you and your mentor have agreed upon roles and responsibilities. In the next section, I provide some ways to help ensure a successful mentorship relationship.

# How Do I Work With a Board of Mentors?

An essential component to the mentoring process is defining the roles and responsibilities of both the mentor and the mentee. In the previous section, I described characteristics that you should seek in a mentor. Similarly, there are actions and behaviors for which the mentee is responsible to ensure an effective mentoring relationship and project success. Key responsibilities (Macrina, 2014) for mentees include:

- Taking lead in planning and goal setting
- Completing agreed-upon responsibilities
- Completing responsibilities in a timely manner
- Scheduling and meeting regularly with the mentor
- Being respectful and appreciative of the mentor, including the mentor's time
- Maintaining meeting notes
- Sharing all relevant project information and progress with the mentor
- Conducting research in full compliance with the approved IRB study protocol
- Fully disclosing competing interests that might create a real or perceived conflict of interest in relationship to the mentor's or mentee's research

The roles and responsibilities of both the mentor and mentee should be determined in a collaborative manner and agreed upon by both individuals.

Other mentoring parameters that should be discussed and agreed upon include the project timeline, anticipated length of the mentoring relationship, how project information will be shared, how authorship (if applicable) will be determined, and how the mentorship relationship will be evaluated to determine if it is a positive experience for both the mentor and mentee and if changes need to be made. Worksheet 5-1 includes a mentorship agreement table you may use to help guide this process.

# Summary

Conducting clinical education research can be an exciting and rewarding endeavor, despite the process being complex and multifaceted. One step you can take to optimize your success and the success of the project is to create a board of mentors. A board of mentors can offer you support across multiple areas pertinent to your research project. It is important to identify mentors that will be supportive, involved, and treat you as a respected collaborator, among other characteristics. For each mentorship relationship, you will need to work with your mentor to establish roles and responsibilities for each of you. With a well-designed, supportive board of mentors you will have the great potential for conducting rigorous and meaningful clinical education research.

# References

American Academy of Physician Associates. (n.d.). AAPA-PAEA research fellowship. https://www.aapa.org/research/aapa-paea-research-fellowship/

American Physical Therapy Association Academy of Research. (n.d.). Evidence-based practice sig. *MemberClicks*. Retrieved August 1, 2022, from https://aptr.memberclicks.net/evidence-based-practice-sig

American Speech-Language-Hearing Association. (n.d.). Researcher resources. *American Speech-Language-Hearing Association*. Retrieved August 1, 2022, from https://www.asha.org/research/researcher-resources/

Disrupting Academic Bullying. (n.d.). Retrieved April 1, 2022, from https://www.graduate.ombudsman.vt.edu/disrupting_academic_bullying.html

Gewin, V. (2021, May 11). How to blow the whistle on an academic bully. *Nature News*. Retrieved August 1, 2022, from https://www.nature.com/articles/d41586-021-01252-z

Macrina, F. L. (2014). *Scientific integrity: Text and cases in responsible conduct of research*. John Wiley & Sons.

Nakamura, J., & Shernoff, D. J. (2009). *Good mentoring: Fostering excellent practice in higher education*. Jossey-Bass.

# Worksheet 5-1:
# Board of Mentors

**Mentoring Planning**

| Project Title: |
| --- |
| Research Question: |

| Areas of Needed Support | Potential Mentors |
| --- | --- |
| 1. | a.<br>b.<br>c. |
| 2. | a.<br>b.<br>c. |
| 3. | a.<br>b.<br>c. |
| 4. | a.<br>b.<br>c. |
| 5. | a.<br>b.<br>c. |
| 6. | a.<br>b.<br>c. |
| 7. | a.<br>b.<br>c. |
| 8. | a.<br>b.<br>c. |
| 9. | a.<br>b.<br>c. |
| 10. | a.<br>b.<br>c. |

*(continued)*

# Worksheet 5-1:
# Board of Mentors (continued)

**Mentorship Agreement**

| | |
|---|---|
| Mentee Name: | Mentor Name: |

Project Title:

Anticipated Project Timeline:

Frequency and Mode of Meetings:

Will the project result in presentations and/or publications?      Yes      No
If yes, how will authorship be determined?

Areas of Support:
    a.

    b.

    c.

    d.

Notes on Project Progress:

Date to Update Mentorship Agreement:

*(continued)*

# Worksheet 5-1:
# Board of Mentors (continued)

**Who Is on Your Board of Mentors?**

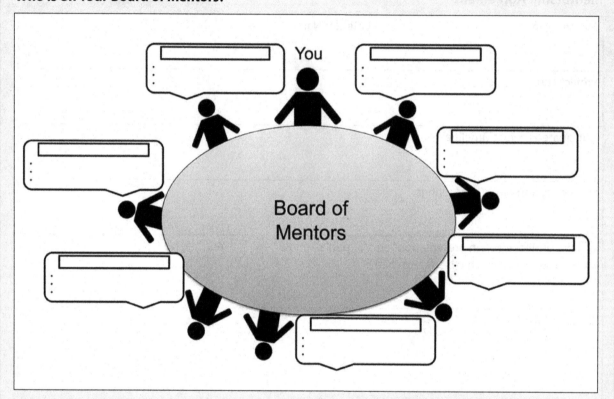

# Quantitative Research Foundational Concepts

*Jessica Brown, PhD, CCC-SLP*

As you looked through the table of contents for this book, I bet the chapter on quantitative research was the one you were most interested in skipping. If that's the case, I wouldn't blame you. When I decided that I wanted my career to focus on clinical practices, education, and research, I quickly realized it unfortunately meant I would have to acquire skills and knowledge in statistics—eek! At times, the road felt like a long, dry, boring walk through the Saharan desert. However, I soon began to realize that without a strong foundation in quantitative design and analysis, I would be unable to answer the important clinical questions that kept my mind racing at night. Skip forward almost 20 years later and I can say that designing research and selecting statistical analyses that match my clinical goals is actually an exciting process (no, seriously!).

But you're probably thinking … sure, exciting for you, but you are a nerd and pursued a career in research. And if you're thinking that, you're right! (And we use *nerd* in a kind and loving way!) However, the need and desire for performing research is not isolated to the academic nerds. Something I quickly realized when I started my educational career was the divide between research labs and providers

(e.g., hospitals, schools, clinics, skilled nursing facilities). What was even worse was morphing into an academic faculty member and experiencing first-hand the wide, desolate valleys that *can* (but don't always) exist between research faculty, clinical faculty, and students. Nerd or not, we all have the ability and responsibility to fill those gaps and caulk those divides to improve clinical practices and clinical education. In fact, almost every profession in the world demands it and seeks to incorporate some version of an evidence-based practice triad into its guidelines and practices. The question we are faced with now is how to marry and merge the best scientific evidence, clinical expertise, and patient value components of evidence-based practice into clinical education. I believe the answer is simple—quantitative research regarding clinical and educational practices performed by actual clinicians and educators (gasp!). The evidence-based education model (Ginsberg et al., 2012) takes this concept a step further to specify that in clinical education, we must triangulate information regarding the scholarship of teaching and learning, instructor-learner interaction, and pedagogical content knowledge to make decisions regarding best practices.

DeRuiter, M., & Ginsberg, S. M. (Eds.). *Clinician's Guide to Applying, Conducting, and Disseminating Clinical Education Research* (pp. 59-79).

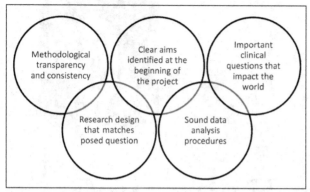

**Figure 6-1.** Characteristics of quantitative research design.

So, why quantitative research? Maybe you've never considered yourself a *researcher* or never thought about conducting research. But guess what? You already do it every single day when you help your students make unique, person-centered clinical decisions and you yourself plan and adjust your educational practices. The difference between the *you's* and the *me's*? Intention! For the rest of this chapter, the goal will be to provide advice and ideas on how to formalize the research process within your clinical education practices. Whether your questions are about the assessment and treatment provided by students to clients, the advancement of knowledge within students in a given semester, or even about your successful techniques as a clinical educator, quantitative research can help provide those answers through (somewhat) painless embedment into your day-to-day practices.

# Research Design Considerations

In other chapters of this book, my co-authors will provide advice on developing research questions, creating sound research studies, and many more details into the nuances of research design in clinical education. We are in a bit of a chicken-egg situation. If you find yourself wanting to first consider your research questions and then consider how to match it to a quantitative method, feel free to skip ahead and come back to this chapter later. If you find yourself interested in learning about the research design possibilities before you narrow down a particular question, keep on reading. We will start with some generalities to consider as you dive into quantitative methods.

## General Decisions to Be Made

### Is Quantitative Research Right for Me?

Quantitative research refers to systematic methods of gathering and analyzing data (primarily numerical) to answer predetermined questions and test hypotheses.

Successful implementation of quantitative methods requires that the individual performing the research consider and achieve a variety of key components in their design and implementation (Figure 6-1; Duckett, 2021). Although this is not an exhaustive list of features that contribute to quantitative research, acknowledging the global characteristics of these methods prior to research implementation can enhance research outcomes. Achieving each of these aims can certainly happen when working alone; however, establishing a team of individuals, as described in Chapter 5, to assist with idea development, identification of design flaws, consistency in methodology, and integrity of statistical analyses will ensure that these key components can easily be incorporated. See Chapter 5 for developing your own board of mentors who can be helpful.

When considering quantitative research in clinical education, many factors can influence your ultimate decisions. If your questions about clinical education research or current methodologies don't match some of the factors listed in Figure 6-1, quantitative research may not be the appropriate route to follow. Conversely, you may need to make some adjustments to your design before diving in. As stated before, other chapters in this book will help you to unpack the necessities for different components in Figure 6-1. For now, we will focus on methodological options that align with quantitative research, as well as some data analysis procedures that you may wish to pursue in alignment with your collection methods and obtained data.

## Variables

A variable is the "thing" you intend to study. Some of those variables are constant and controlled throughout the research study by you, in other words, the intervention you are implementing. These consistent variables are called *independent variables*. Think of these as the cause or reason that a particular outcome might occur. The independent variable is manipulated by the researcher to test an outcome. Conversely, *dependent variables* are those that you are measuring to evaluate whether something has happened. Think of these as your effect (e.g., student knowledge regarding a clinical construct, SOAP [subjective, objective, assessment, plan] note proficiency). At its core, these numbers and data that you gather depend on the independent variable in your study. It is vital to *operationally define* your variables prior to initiating a study. Having clear, detailed explanations of your variables will allow you to study a cause and effect with certainty. Your variables should be defined clearly enough that another researcher without intimate knowledge of your study could replicate the methods simply by reading your operational definitions. Let's take the example of "SOAP note proficiency" that I used before. Imagine you are wondering whether your feedback format, components, or frequency to students are impacting their proficiency in documentation using the SOAP note method. You have developed an amazing and novel way to provide student feedback on their writing that you are sure will influence their success with astounding statistical significance. The only problem is evaluating writing is subjective. Your definition of "proficiency" may be far different from my definition. Therefore, ratings and feedback from one clinical educator may differ vastly from another. The answer? Operationally define your variable such that there is no question about how you view proficiency. In this example, maybe you have a very clear rubric that is created before you begin the semester. Each component of the SOAP note is specifically laid out on the rubric with defined requirements of achievement for each rubric rating. You have worked with other team members to create multiple rubric drafts, have piloted the rubric with various students and clinical educators, and are confident that you have a sound and consistent operational definition of proficiency. In this case, you are ready to gather a baseline (more to come on that in a minute) and let the amazing and novel feedback methodology begin! You also have a clear idea of your independent and dependent variables and can provide transparent and consistent definitions to consider beginning your research study.

### Reliability

The terms reliability and validity are likely ones that you have heard before. Broadly, these concepts define the psychometric properties of various research instruments. *Reliability* refers to the consistency with which the research was conducted and the results were obtained. For example, these measures could relate to consistency of collected data between time points (i.e., test-retest reliability) or among raters (i.e., interrater reliability). Focus on different types of reliability may be relevant depending on your research aims and methods. For example, intervention provision and data collection from one individual team member removes the potential confound of interrater reliability concerns.

### Validity

*Validity* refers to the strength of a research instrument to meet its intended aims; in other words, does the tool do what it was designed to do? As with reliability, various forms of validity exist and must be considered when designing and implementing research studies. Of particular importance in clinical education research is the concept of clinical validity (i.e., relatedness to a clinical outcome) or social validity (i.e., importance or acceptability of goals and outcomes). Similar to the concept of ecological validity, these terms encompass the extent to which the findings or results can be generalized to real-world settings and of functional, substantial importance to a group of individuals. The consideration is whether, and to what extent, the research you intend to perform and the results you obtain

reflect and inform clinical education. External validity is a similar construct and relates to the degree to which the research can be generalized to other settings. Are the results obtained in your research only relatable to the students and clinical experiences that you studied, or can the results be broadly applied across individuals and contexts? Internal validity is most closely tied with the decision made prior to and while conducting your research. Internal validity reflects whether the research methods can answer posed questions and hypotheses without bias or influence from confounding, outside variables. Ascertaining whether your observed outcomes are due to the independent variable or to additional factors reflects the extent of your study's internal validity. These concepts will require deep reflection and foresight when designing and initiating quantitative research methodologies.

# SINGLE-SUBJECT RESEARCH DESIGN

In my opinion, single-subject design is the creme de la creme of clinical education research. Other researchers agree with me. In a 2010 paper, Johnston and Smith noted that "a new level of understanding is needed to harness the power of SSDs [single-subject design] to advance the science supporting [health] fields" (p. 4). These types of studies are perfectly suited for initial evaluations of an intervention's potential effectiveness when more robust experimental design options are neither feasible nor reasonable to pursue. Despite being widely used, single-subject design methods may be overlooked in modern research discussions and education. But don't let that fool you. The methods discussed later may be some of the most vital to inform future disciplinary research and clinical education practices. So, let's dive in. In 2010, What Works Clearinghouse (WWC) published a technical document on single-subject design outlining anything and everything you would want to know about these research methodology options (Kratochwill et al., 2010). Within those guidelines, they determined and discussed a set of single-case design standards by which such studies should be judged. These standards included three important steps to design, implementation, and evaluation of single-case research (Figure 6-2). The first step is a judgment regarding the study design itself—that is, does the research design meet evidence standards and include necessary components that we previously discussed, including but not limited to operational definitions of independent and dependent variables, controlled data collection factoring in external and internal validity, fidelity, and reliability. If determined that a study design meets standards or meets standards with some reservation, the next step requires data visualization and analysis of each outcome variable (more to come on this). Those data that show strong or moderate evidence of treatment effectiveness following visual analysis should be evaluated

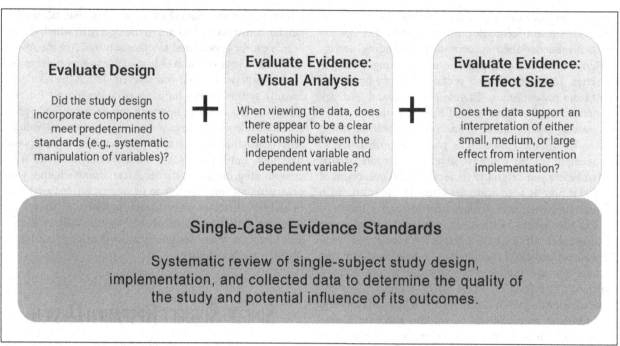

**Figure 6-2.** Single-case research evidence standards.

for determination of effect size, a quantitative measure of the magnitude of effectiveness of a given experiment. In the sections that follow, we will discuss various elements of these standards as you consider how to implement single-subject design into your clinical education practices.

## Defining a Subject or Case

In clinical education research, it is most likely that your *subject* or *case* might be a single student or client. The concept of case study research has no one definition; however, the concept globally relates to in-depth exploration of an event or phenomena in a naturalistic environment rather than a controlled, experimental environment. The term *single-subject design* can further define your research practices within case study research and is most frequently thought of as a systematic observation or evaluation of an individual entity (e.g., person, data point). However, single-subject design options don't have to strictly involve only one person. You could consider your subject to be any kind of single entity—a group of students, a clinical cohort, a class roster, or a treatment group, for example. In this regard, it is important you ensure that each individual person in your study is treated in the exact same manner so you are truly studying the entity in its entirety. The point then is not to look at individual variation but rather to garner information about the subject or group. Keeping these cases small in number will help to reduce the potential variability and outside confounds that could be contributing to the observed change (your dependent variable data). In

fact, single-subject designs are ideal when you don't have a large group of individuals to enroll in a study. Typically, in these cases, you want to compare the individual or entity to themselves. The goal would be to repeatedly collect data regarding your dependent variable using the same method at regularly scheduled intervals. If you wish to incorporate a control group and complete between group comparisons, you are merging into the world of experimental research and beyond the naturalistic environments of case design and single-subject research studies. Although experimental research is often quantitative in nature, the required components of those studies may reach beyond the scope of your intended study goals (e.g., randomized control trials). Finding a friend with expertise in research who can help you flush out your ideas and determine the best methodological fit for your proposed aims will help you determine whether single-subject design is an appropriate option.

## Baseline Data

When starting with single-subject design research, one of the most important things you must do is collect *baseline data* for your dependent variable that you wish to study. The goal is to gain enough information about the frequency, intensity, or duration of a given case/subject's behaviors and trends so that once an intervention phase is implemented you can make meaningful inferences regarding potential relationships between intervention and behavioral changes. Gathering baseline data can be considered as your very own control group before you make a change or introduce the independent variable. Most research experts will tell you that a minimum of three baseline data points should be gathered prior to initiating an intervention. The WWC standards recommend a baseline of five data points (Kratochwill et al., 2010). In an ideal world, you would collect the three recommended baseline data points and see a completely stable profile—that is, little to no variation in the dependent variable you are measuring and no increasing or decreasing data trends. The subject's or case's behavior will fall within a predictable, small range of numbers for which you can say with certainty is their typical performance without intervention. For example, a subject's baseline scores on a handwriting rubric fall between 3 and 4 points (out of 10) on three separate occasions prior to initiating occupational therapy interventions. Gaining a stable baseline is important as this data will be used as your true north, the comparison values to later determine the effectiveness of your intervention. Without this comparison, interpreting your treatment would be impossible.

I would be lying if I told you that every single-subject design study I've ever done started with a stable and beautiful baseline data profile. Humans aren't always built that way. So, what can a person do? We've already established that if you move forward with the study without a stable baseline, it may cause difficulties later when attempting to analyze or interpret your data and draw meaningful conclusions. If necessary, you may need to extend the baseline portion of your study for a longer period of time. Collecting a few more data points beyond the recommended three to five may help you to see a more stable trend that would allow you to feel comfortable in moving forward with the study. The other solution to this problem might lie within your research methods themselves. It is possible that you lack control in the study and that additional external variables are contributing to baseline performance on the dependent variable. In that case, brainstorming additional methods to tighten your data collection procedures and reduce the influence of confounds may be appropriate before moving forward. Unfortunately, and fortunately, research is all about trial and error.

## The A and B of Single-Subject Design

For whatever reason, someone a long time ago decided that single-subject design should be categorized by the "A" and "B" *phases*. We will also provide some examples of when a "C" phase comes into play. For those of us who are novices to the research world, this actually works out quite well. For each letter assigned to a particular part of your research (the phase), you can clearly conceptualize what is being done, by whom, that you intend to evaluate. The case or subject would be exposed to one phase (independent variable) at a time. In these designs, the decision to switch between phases occurs because of trends in data

or behaviors demonstrated by your subject rather than at fixed intervals. Oftentimes, this occurs when your dependent variable demonstrates little variability. Consistent with recommendations regarding baseline data collection, standards set forth by WWC (Kratochwill et al., 2010) designate that a research phase should include at least five data points to allow for sufficient measurement of level, trend, and variability to derive meaningful evaluations of causal relationships. Let me explain possible variations in phase implementation for single-subject design a bit further. Please note that the designs described further in the following are the basic and most common options utilized in single-subject design. However, variations of these methods are available if maximally suited for your particular question and case.

### A-B Design

Let's say that you plan to start a new training method with your clinical students. You have been doing some "business as usual" work with them during the semester and are about to start something brand new. Well, your A phase would be your baseline—the performance of your students given the business-as-usual treatment before you start the super special new educational method. As soon as you begin implementing the new component, you are in the B phase. The goal is to then see what, if any, changes in student performance can be gleaned. Theoretically, you can then say that any change in performance on a particular construct (either positive or negative) may likely be due to the implementation of the new educational method. Figure 6-3 visually depicts an A-B design with the new intervention beginning in week 4 of the semester. As depicted in this graph, the subject had a baseline performance in the first 3 weeks that was relatively stable (between three and four). Once the intervention phase begins, you may notice that continued implementation resulted in increased student achievement across the entirety of the semester with relative consistency in advancing performance trends.

You may wish to choose an A-B design if you are looking for a relatively quick and easy study to implement. A-B designs are appropriate to provide some basic and rudimentary evidence for determining whether you may want to further pursue an intervention or line of research. In other words, A-B designs may be considered as precursors to additional experimental studies you wish to perform. A downside of an A-B design is that you may not be able to clearly and definitively say that the intervention (independent variable) was responsible for the change in your dependent variable. It is possible that outside of confounding factors are also influencing performance and your study lacks internal validity. Therefore, you may want to consider an A-B-A design when possible. We will talk about this strategy next.

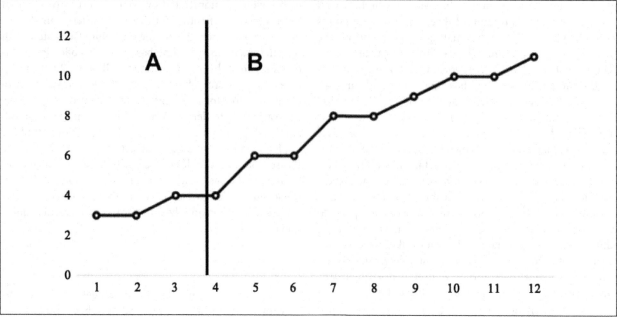

**Figure 6-3.** A-B single-subject research design.

---

# Box 6-1:
## Example of A-B-A Design

Let's unpack an example. You are noticing that students are struggling to tie the lesson plan components to the intervention methods or constructs in their sessions. You have created a method where students answer questions regarding these concepts and the relationship between their activity and the clinical construct. Through these questions/answers, you are able to gather data regarding their clinical knowledge. You notice that despite continually teaching and giving feedback to students, you are not seeing an increase in their success on the question/answer activities. Therefore, you decide it might be beneficial to create the lesson plan yourself for a few weeks. Your hope is that by creating activities that fully match the intended clinical construct, your students will implicitly learn and grow in their knowledge and skills. After 6 weeks of your lesson planning, you want to see if students improve (or maintain improvement) when they switch back to creating lesson plans themselves. Figure 6-4 visually depicts the A-B-A design with implementation of supervisor-created lesson plans in week 6 and student-created lesson plans in weeks 12 and beyond. You may notice in this example that students' knowledge improved when the supervisor began creating lesson plans (end of initial phase A and start of phase B). When phase A was again initiated, knowledge scores were not as high as they were toward the end of phase B (intervention phase); however, maintenance of this knowledge and skills were still evident.

You may wish to choose an A-B-A design if you are again looking for ease and feasibility of implementation. These studies are well suited for treatments that are expected to have large and somewhat immediate effects on a subject or case. These are also suited for behaviors that are truly dependent on a particular treatment or intervention. A downside to reversal design is that not all behaviors are reversible. Sometimes, by implementing an intervention (particularly with a human student), you take the chance that you have changed their behavior forever. It is possible their newly learned skill supplement to the intervention is now with them and cannot be taken away. In this case, the second A phase may not in fact confirm your findings. Clearly thinking about the likelihood of a behavior's ability to be present or absent solely based on the intervention will be important before implementing an A-B-A design. Figure 6-4 demonstrates a reversal design.

---

## A-B-A Design

Now you are trying to get fancy and are implementing what is known as a *reversal design*. You believe that your brand-spanking-new idea for clinical education is going to be absolutely amazing. But you also hypothesize that student performance may only increase or decrease (depending on what you hope/expect it to do) while you are actually implementing your new idea. You aren't sure if those same effects will be maintained after you stop implementing your idea, but you know it would be worthwhile

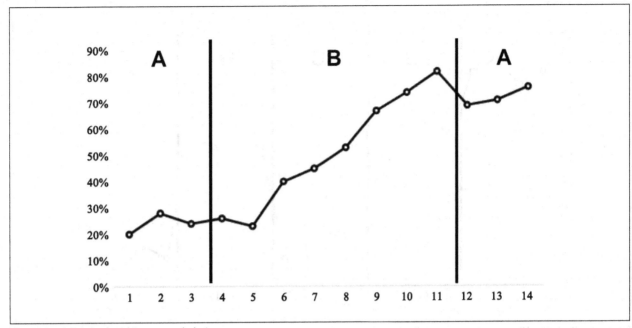

**Figure 6-4.** A-B-A single-subject research design.

to find out. You also want to be really sure that no other factors are influencing your subject's performance. Therefore, you are reluctant to introduce a simple A-B design. In other words, you are a research design rock star and are looking for the most interval validity you can get. If you notice that a behavior changes once a B phase is implemented and changes back closer to baseline when the intervention is not present (second A), you can say with good certainty that the intervention was responsible for the behavior change. Note that oftentimes what we mean as reversal is simply a withdrawal or taking away of the intervention.

## Alternating Treatment Designs

In an *alternating treatment design*, you are doing just as the name implies—switching back and forth between treatments and looking at the change in your dependent variable. Each phase of the design then is a different treatment. This could look something like A-B-C-B-C-A. Or something crazy like that. In this example, you are looking at global baseline measures (A) before and after treatment implementation, but you are switching between two different treatments (B and C) during the intervention phases. Such a method could be very beneficial to determining which of the two interventions has a greater effect on behavior but only if the change in behavior is expected to be quick—that is, when your treatment is fast.

Figure 6-5 visually depicts an alternating treatment design for a behavior that you wish to see decrease during the intervention phases. The research design represents an A-B-C-B-C design with a change in phase every four sessions.

## Box 6-2: Example of A-B-C-B-C-A Design

Your question at the end of the study might be to determine which of the interventions were more successful at decreasing the negative behavior. Let's pretend that the undesirable behavior is negative self-talk from students during your meetings (e.g., "I don't know, this is too hard, I will never understand this"). Of course, we will have operationally defined what we deem as negative self-talk before study implementation. But you believe that one of two potential methods might influence student behavior. One intervention relies on shutting down the negative talk during your twice-weekly meetings with the students. You start students off with 50 dinner place setting pictures at the beginning of the semester. For each time a student says something negative about themselves, you will take away a picture. If a student loses all their pictures, they won't get to partake in the fancy year-end dinner you are hosting for your student cohort. The other intervention requires the student to self-reflect on their strengths and challenges in a notebook right before the weekly supervisor meeting. You wonder if providing a safe space for students to note their self-perceived flaws and doubts, as well as their accomplishments, gets them in a good head space and decreases the frequency of negative self-talk during meetings. Under the alternating treatment design approach, you decide to switch between these two interventions every other week. Again, the goal is to determine which approach is more effective at decreasing negative self-talk. Beware, however, of a tricky thing called *maturation* that we will discuss a little later in the chapter.

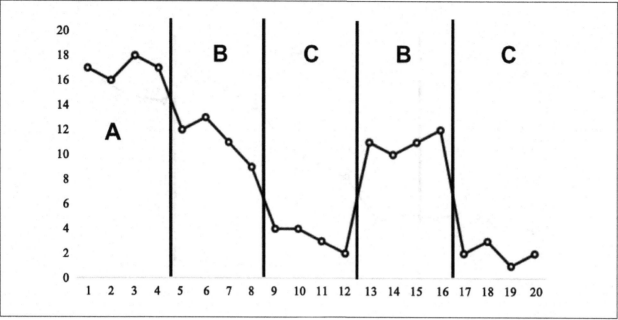

**Figure 6-5.** Alternating treatment single-subject design.

## Multiple Baseline Design

I mentioned earlier that one potential problem with reversal designs is that a behavior may in fact not be reversible. Your intervention may have a lasting impact on the case or subject. Another potential challenge of these designs relates to ethics. If you implement an intervention and see that it's causing a change in your dependent variable in a desired or improved direction, it may in fact be unethical to later withhold that treatment to collect A phase or baseline data. For example, if you developed a clinical education strategy that when done regularly reduces student stress, anxiety, and likelihood of burnout, it would be problematic to take that intervention away. The good news is that we have a solution to these two problems known as *multiple baseline design*. In a multiple baseline design, two or more behaviors are assessed during the baseline data collection phase. An intervention is begun to hopefully alter one of the behaviors while the other remains unaffected. After time has elapsed, the intervention is then applied to the other behavior. There are different versions of a multiple baseline design approach. Globally, these types of single-subject design studies are intended to gradually and incrementally introduce new phases and interventions to the same subject or case (or even for multiple cases or settings). Multiple baseline designs are ideal because they do not require you to withdraw any type of intervention. Because of this, they are well suited for those behaviors that are not reversible. Some ethical considerations must be taken when using multiple baseline designs if you keep individuals or behaviors out of a particular treatment for an extended period of time. You can argue, however, that all individuals or behaviors in the study will ultimately be exposed to the treatment. Confused? How about some examples.

Let's start with considering providing an intervention to a group of students but each at different starting times. You would begin your study by collecting baseline data on all participants at the same time. After gaining a steady baseline for Participant 1 (three total baseline sessions), you would implement the intervention phase of your study. However, you would wait to begin a treatment phase for Participants 2 and 3 and instead continue to collect baseline data. After time, you would add the intervention for Participant 2 while continuing to collect baseline data for Participant 3—and so on. In this example, let's imagine that you started intervention for Participant 2 in session five and Participant 3 in session eight. The idea here is that a change in behavior for one participant at the start of an intervention could be coincidence. But if the same trend is noted for three participants at various time points (for example) you can say with great certainty that the intervention was the likely cause. Figure 6-6 demonstrates a multiple baseline design across several participants.

I also mentioned that multiple baseline designs could be created around a single participant or subject but with more than one dependent variable. The idea here being that you are looking at the impact of intervention of more than one behavior. As an example, say your new clinical student is struggling with both the *time* it takes to create a lesson plan, as well as the *quality* of the lesson plan. For a while now, you have been toying with the idea of a goal-setting intervention that you think might be able to impact both of your student's ineffective behaviors. You begin by collecting steady baseline data on both behaviors. Once that is reached, you decide to tackle the quality component because you deem that as most clinically important. You implement your goal-setting intervention and begin to track quality change while still monitoring baseline for the time variable. As the clinical placement progresses, you decide to implement your goal-setting intervention for the time component as well. If you see a change in both of your dependent variables secondary to the introduction of your goal-setting intervention, then it looks like you have a winner!

## Data Visualization

Now that you have some idea of potential options available in single-subject design research and have collected all of your amazing data, you need to figure out what to do with it. A very key component to single-subject design is *data visualization*. You'll hear me talk about this again later when we discuss some global data analysis procedures in quantitative research. But let me make myself very clear—data visualization will be your absolute best friend. Graphs, charts, tables: They can all "show" you things about your data that looking strictly at the numbers often can't. I wouldn't have ever considered myself a right-brained visual person. In fact, brain games that require spatial reasoning are my mortal enemy. However, the value of representing numbers and content in a visual manner is priceless to not only understanding and interpreting your data but also disseminating it to the rest of the world. In single-subject design research, it is most common to create line graphs where the y-axis represents the behavior or dependent variable and the x-axis often represents time indicating various data collection points during each study phase. As shown in many of the previous examples, further inclusion of labels for study phases can enhance the linear data graphing. The goal of data visualization is to help you interpret *level/ rate*, *trends (slope)*, and *variability* within phases of your single-subject designs (Engel & Schutt, 2016). Additional considerations of *immediacy of effect (latency)*, *overlap*, and *statistical effect size calculations* can further elucidate your findings.

## Data Evaluation and Interpretation in Single-Subject Research

Data visualization efforts provided a crucial initial step to evaluating and interpreting data collected in single-subject research design. However, various statistical and descriptive methods are available and likely necessary in sound research design (Byiers et al., 2012). The methods discussed in the following sections highlight commonly used tools for understanding and analyzing your collected data, as well as interpreting intervention outcomes. These features or methods can be used individually, or ideally, collectively, to examine patterns in data within and between phases. Figure 6-7 provides visual examples of the analysis tools described next.

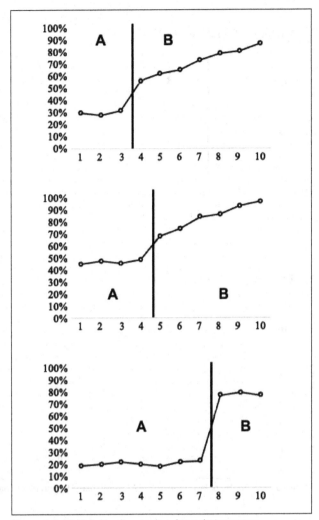

**Figure 6-6.** Multiple baseline single-subject design across participants.

## Level (Rate, Figure 6-7, Panel A)

Likely the most basic component of visual inspection, changes in *level* relate to any noticeable difference (increase or decrease) in the data points between the non-intervention and intervention phases of the study. If the dependent variable is much higher or lower in an intervention phase, one can assume that the treatment had an effect. The example in Figure 6-7 depicts a large, increased change in rate or level following completion of phase A (baseline phase) and initiation of phase B (intervention phase).

## Trend (Slope, Figure 6-7, Panel B)

*Trend* refers to a gradual decrease or increase in the dependent variable across the course of the intervention. It is possible that a given behavior or skill may not

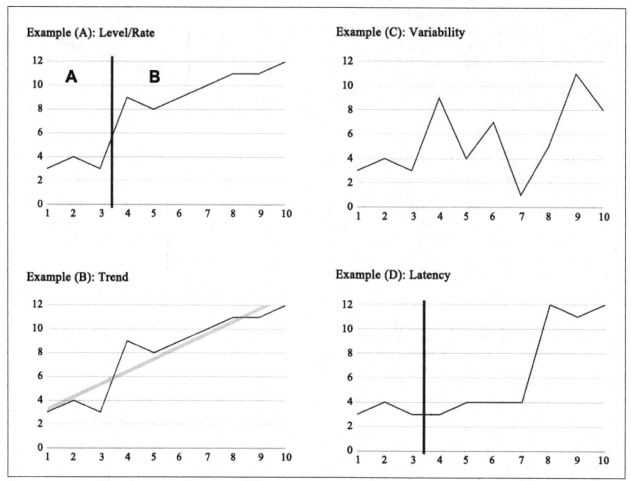

**Figure 6-7.** Examples of level/rate (panel A), trend (panel B), variability (panel C), and latency (panel D).

immediately change upon introduction of an intervention phase. Thus, distinct observations of level may not be as clear. However, an increase or decrease within a phase that differs from baseline performance can be compelling when determining whether or not an intervention had an effect. Numerically, inclusion of *trend lines* (visual depiction of a prevailing pattern of performance) and evaluation of the *slope* (indicating rate of change) of graphed data points can assist in understanding the magnitude of a given trend. The example in Figure 6-7 depicts an overall increasing trend visible by the added thick, gray trend line.

## Variability
## (Figure 6-7, Panel C)

The concept of *variability* refers to how different or discrepant the data points are within a single phase. High variability in either a baseline or intervention phase makes interpretation of the intervention effect more difficult. A lack of stability in performance during a given phase could be explained by a great number of potential factors, both related and unrelated to the variables of interest. Drawing range lines on graphed data or documenting range values

when interpreting research outcomes can illuminate the extent to which variability contributed to intervention effectiveness. The example in Figure 6-7 depicts a highly unstable performance with a great deal of variability. Data across points range from 1 to 11 and are inconsistent across the course of the study.

## Latency
## (Immediacy of Effect, Figure 6-7, Panel D)

*Latency* refers to the amount of time it takes for a dependent variable to change once a phase or change in condition is initiated. If a change occurs shortly after introduction of an intervention, it is likely that the intervention itself was effective and responsible for the change. The example in Figure 6-7 depicts a longer latency such that the effect of the intervention is not noticeable until data point 8 despite the intervention being applied following data point 3. Given this long latency for change, it is possible that additional confounding factors are influencing performance within the measured dependent variable and the change may not be attributable to the provided intervention.

## Overlap

Comparing the data points collected during a baseline or non-intervention phase vs. an intervention phase can help to glean information about the impact of the intervention. The presence of little to no *overlap* between phase data allows you to infer that the intervention had a substantial impact on the evaluated behavior or skill. Calculating the percentage of non-overlapping data (PND; Scruggs et al., 1987) can provide insight into the magnitude of your intervention's effects. The greater the PND the greater the impact or effect of the intervention on the dependent variable. In words that people can actually understand, the less data points that overlap, the better! PND is calculated by determining the percentage of data points during intervention phases that exceed the highest (or lowest) data point during the baseline or nonintervention phase. If you are hoping that an intervention has a negative result on a behavior, or results in a decrease in a given construct, you would count how many data points during your intervention phase (B) are below the lowest data point in your baseline phase (A). You would take that calculated number and divide it by the total number of collected data points in your intervention phase.

---

### Box 6-3: Calculating the Percentage of Non-Overlapping Data

Let's take an example and imagine that in your baseline or non-intervention phase, the lowest data point you collected had a value of 25. During your intervention phase, you calculated a total of 10 data points. When you looked at your data, 6 of the 10 data points fell below the value of 25; therefore, your PND would be calculated by calculating 6 divided by 10 equaling 60%.

---

## Effect Size: Tau-U

Visual analysis of data in isolation does not allow for statistical interpretation of data trends in single-subject research design. Although useful, incorporating inferential methods that objectively calculate the potential impact of an intervention is advantageous (Maggin & Chafouleas, 2013; Parker et al., 2011a). These calculations are known as *effect size* calculations. Effect size refers to the amount or meaningfulness of the relationship between two items. For example, is the observed change in your data related to your intervention in a statistically meaningful manner? Use of such measures allows you to add objectivity to evaluation of your data rather than relying solely on the somewhat subjective visualization components previously described. Two measures of effect size in single-subject research are

particularly useful. The first is Tau-U, a method unique to single-subject designs. This method combines information regarding performance trend within phases along with non-overlap between phases to derive statistical assumptions about the impact of a given intervention (Lee & Cherney, 2018). This method may be particularly useful when visual inspection alone is insufficient in determining the influence of an intervention. Tau-U is also beneficial in circumstances when a trend in baseline data was noted (Parker et al., 2011b).

## Effect Size: Standardized Mean Difference

Standardized mean difference is a computation of effect size that is widely used in communication sciences and disorders research and particularly in single-subject design. To complete this calculation, the difference between the mean (average) performance in the baseline and intervention phase is calculated and subsequently divided by the standard deviation of the baseline phase (Busk & Serlin, 1992). The resultant value can be interpreted using a traditional Cohen's *d* statistic (Fritz et al., 2012) and interpreted as the extent to which the level between two phases is or is not significant.

## *Additional Considerations in Single-Subject Research*

As we wrap up this overview of single-subject research, I would be remiss not to mention some potential pitfalls commonly occurring with these types of research designs. Understanding the likelihood of such pitfalls and generating alternate options prior to beginning a study may save you a great deal of time and energy in the end. Three that I will focus on include influence of repeated testing, maintenance and generalization, and history and maturation.

## Repeated Testing Effects

Within the cognitive literature, there is a great deal of support for contextualized and naturalistic training opportunities. Supporters of these training methods (me included) purport that learning of behaviors is maximally beneficial when done within the setting and context that you will need to use a behavior. Important to this clinical practice is that the potential for repeated testing effects to influence outcomes are great. What I mean by that is the process of completing a particular task (e.g., taking a test, practicing a set of stimuli) results in improvement on that particular task. It does *not* necessarily mean that an individual has improved globally in the construct you are measuring within the context in which they will need that behavior. Confused? I like using the example of science and a dog.

Catching a frisbee requires a complex understanding of a variety of types of science ... geometry, physics, anatomy. My dog can practice catching a frisbee repeatedly and he may become so adept that he is suitable for enrollment in a national contest. But just because he is amazing at catching a frisbee does not mean that he has in fact grasped the complexities of geometry, physics, and anatomy. My point? Be careful that the subject does not demonstrate a particular behavior or response simply because they are learning how to "take the test." In other words, repeated exposure to your data collection method or activity itself may in fact influence and change performance. Including collection of maintenance and generalization data within your research design may help to account for potential repeated testing influences.

## Maintenance and Generalization

Two concepts in single-subject research design can be implemented with relative ease and contribute positively to the interpretation of your findings–that is, maintenance and generalization. *Generalization* measures refer to data collection on constructs similar to your dependent variable of study but with stimuli that are untrained. In clinical education research, you could imagine that you are working on an intervention to support a systematic, procedural approach to decision making when a student is presented with a case study. You would like to know if your treatment methods can generalize or extend to cases that were not specifically taught or practiced within your intervention. Presenting a student with an untrained case and measuring their success relative to your dependent variables would represent their ability to generalize skills learned during intervention to untrained stimuli. This would allow you to determine the extent to which your intervention was clinically and educationally meaningful for the student beyond study participation. *Maintenance* data collection is similar in that your goal is to determine how long the effects of an intervention will last beyond the intervention phase. You may wish to retest or re-assess behaviors days, weeks, or months following intervention to determine the potential for lasting impacts of learned behaviors or skills once the intervention phase has lapsed.

## History and Maturation

Participant history and maturation are two important elements in interpreting single-subject data. *History* refers to events or components of a participant's life that co-occur with research involvement and potentially impact results. History is an important potential threat to single-subject research, as this type of data collection occurs over time. Imagine that you are examining the effects of a novel clinical education method for a first-year student while they are simultaneously participating in content classes aimed at teaching similar information. In this example, it would be impossible to derive whether it was the novel clinical education methods or education from content courses that impacted student behavior. Single-subject research design that incorporates phase repetition (e.g., A-B-A-B designs) or those that seek to eliminate outside influence (e.g., ensuring a clinical rotation is the only education a student receives in a given subject) may help to reduce some uncertainty when interpreting results. *Maturation* refers to naturally occurring changes within a participant over time. Given that data in single-subject designs are collected over days, weeks, months, or even years, it is plausible to assume that the subject being observed will change in their skill set or behaviors. Including additional control (baseline) phases or increasing frequency of repeated data measurement within the experiment may provide insight into natural maturation behaviors within a participant.

# SURVEY RESEARCH

When I started conducting research, I mistakenly saw survey studies as the "low-hanging fruit." I assumed it was easy to type up any old questions I had, ask people to answer those questions on paper or electronically, and ultimately gain rich, valuable data that would change clinical practice and education as we know it. Although this is certainly a possibility in the clinical education world, survey design requires careful thought and planning in order to work effectively. With some foresight and a pinch of help from a magic ball, survey design can be a treasure trove of data collection. Let's talk about how to make that happen. As cited by Kraemer (1991), survey research includes three distinguishing components (Figure 6-8), which when considered adequately, can facilitate the answering of important questions or solving of critical problems relative to your research purpose. One must understand and acknowledge the purpose of survey research overall and the clear purpose of distinct survey methods when designing a study of this nature.

## *Survey Purpose*

Survey research methodologies can provide rich information to compliment other data sources. Many studies that I have performed include traditional quantitative data methods, as well as self-reported information by populations of interest either through survey or qualitative research methods (more to come on that in the next chapter of this book). The information gained from survey research may not be feasibly gained by other methods. Consider the resources in time and finances that it might take to interview professionals around the country or the world. Creation of a survey that includes various question types

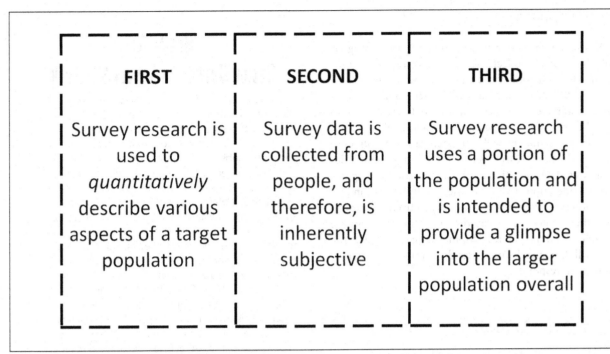

| FIRST | SECOND | THIRD |
| --- | --- | --- |
| Survey research is used to *quantitatively* describe various aspects of a target population | Survey data is collected from people, and therefore, is inherently subjective | Survey research uses a portion of the population and is intended to provide a glimpse into the larger population overall |

**Figure 6-8.** Distinguishing characteristics of survey research.

might allow you to gain a large amount of critical information without the necessity for a large team and lengthy data collection efforts. In other words, surveys have a lot of potential to enhance your research!

The potential standardization of survey methodologies allows for additional advantages. Through completion of a survey, you can ensure that every respondent was presented with the exact same directions and wording for every question posed. Although you cannot ensure that every individual perceived and processed the question in the same manner, you have to some extent increased the internal validity of your research study through this type of standardization. Creating multiple survey drafts, piloting the survey questions with diverse groups of individuals, and seeking feedback regarding survey methodology and questioning prior to implementing the study can further enhance this standardization of data collection.

Various options exist when creating a survey research plan and selecting the type of survey research in which you hope to engage. Prior to beginning, you must make choices regarding your research study that revolve around the population you intend to survey and the type of data you hope to collect. Two major categories of research studies include *cross-sectional* and *longitudinal* studies. Cross-sectional survey studies are intended to collect information that is a snapshot of a population of interest. Data are collected at a single time point from a representative sample of the target cohort. This is probably the most common design and most likely option for consideration when implementing survey research broadly.

In clinical education research, longitudinal survey studies may be an appropriate or ideal option. Such surveys are intended to repeatedly examine a group or a phenomenon over time. In its simplest form, an example of a longitudinal survey may be a single survey designed around learning outcomes and perceptions of communication sciences courses that students repeatedly complete throughout their enrollment in graduate school. Longitudinal surveys come in various forms. *Trend surveys* are chosen in hopes of collecting data from a single population on the same variables over time. Consider an example of a knowledge and skills survey that a clinical instructor repeatedly completes about the same student over the course of a semester. The intent would be to analyze changes in responses over time or data trends. *Cohort surveys* are intended to collect information from the same population repeatedly, although the questions asked and the data collected may differ over time. The goal is to follow the same group of individuals and gain information about behaviors, opinions, or knowledge at various time points. An example of a cohort survey could relate back to the idea of a graduate cohort that is asked their opinions about graduate school at various times throughout their 2-year program. Finally, a *panel survey* includes selecting a small group of qualified individuals who are willing to provide feedback or information about a given construct repeatedly. Panel surveys typically collect data at frequent intervals. For example, this could include a purposeful, selected group of students who are participating in frequent survey completion about a particular educational method utilized in the internal audiology clinic.

## Survey Instrument Design

Realize that the survey instrument or tool you design is simply the means to collect information within your survey research. We all hope that we will send out a call to complete a created survey tool and will quickly receive thousands of complete responses with rich data for us to analyze and disseminate our research. Design choices within your survey instrument will ultimately strongly influence the success of the research. As we talk about potential design options, data collection methods, and question types, a major consideration should be ease of administration and completion from your respondents. Learn from my experiences—the quicker the survey, the easier the questions are to complete, and the potential for incentive to complete the survey will dramatically influence the number of individuals you get to respond.

## Data Collection Method

Today's society is heavily reliant on electronic forms of communication due to their ease and speed of use. Because of that, electronic survey methods may be an obvious choice when initiating a research study. Many platforms exist to assist with creating an electronic survey. Some are public and free to access while others require paid subscriptions or licenses. Subscription-based survey platforms may be advantageous due to increased flexibility in style/look, question type, and design options.

Survey data collection methods have historically included completion options, such as face-to-face, telephone, and paper/mail-based surveys. Time, cost, and personnel resources should be considered when designing research studies that include particular data collection methods. Such methods may require that you have access to personal information about potential participants in order to begin the recruitment process or that potential respondents take the initiative to reach out to you in order to participate in the survey. In addition, face-to-face or telephone interviews may introduce bias from both the individual conducting the survey and the individual responding. When contemplating options, such as paper completion in-person or by mail, the burden on the respondent is high and hopes of collecting lengthy surveys or detailed responses may be limited. As with all research, maintaining focus on your intended study aims and questions will help to determine which type of data collection method is maximally beneficial for your study.

### Question Types to Consider

The way you ask a question in a survey is not only important for data collection and standardization but it will also substantially influence the type of analysis that you can later perform on that particular data. I have learned this

---

## BOX 6-4:
## DESIGN OPTIONS IN SURVEY RESEARCH

Design options for consideration include but are not limited to forced-choice questions (i.e., requiring an individual to respond before moving further along in the survey), conditional logic (i.e., altering presence or absence of subsequent questions based on previously provided answers), and ability to stop/restart survey completion (i.e., begin answering, save answers, and complete at a later time). Furthermore, electronic survey platforms may differ in how respondents access the survey (e.g., each individual receives a unique link to complete the electronic survey vs. a generic link that any respondent can use), which can contribute to widespread recruitment and respondent diversity. In addition to some of the settings mentioned, consideration of data security and respondent anonymity is crucial prior to selecting a survey platform. Depending on the information you intend to collect, you may need a HIPAA- or FERPA-secure system or one that allows for completely anonymous responses (e.g., doesn't collect IP address information). When you initiate a research proposal with the institutional review board at a given location, information about data collection and security requirements will be clearly outlined. You can read more about the institutional review board in Chapter 9. Depending on your employment setting, access to electronic survey platforms may or may not be a possibility; therefore, consideration of additional data collection methods may be necessary.

---

the hard way over and over again in survey research. When creating a survey, I am often working with my team members to focus on why we are asking a question and what we hope to learn from the data. Keeping that in mind will ensure that the questions created will help you in testing your research hypotheses accurately. I can't tell you how many questions I have had to throw out of surveys because I didn't think it through and ask them correctly in the first place (spoiler: it's a lot). The posed question must also be readily understood at the educational and knowledge level of both the surveyor and the respondent. Survey question wording should be concrete and diminish the possibility of alternate interpretations. Biased or influential language within a question should also be avoided. As I have developed my skills as a researcher, or really just learned from my mistakes, I have realized the importance of piloting surveys or individual survey questions to ensure that the question type and wording match my intended data outcome or clinical question. In the sections that follow, we will briefly discuss the two primary types of questions you may wish to choose from when creating a survey: closed-ended questions and open-ended questions.

1. Closed-ended questions: *Closed-ended questions* in surveys are those the respondents are provided choices from which to answer. The questions posed may require a single answer or allow for multiple selections; however, the respondent must select from what is provided by you, the researcher. Think of this type as the traditional multiple-choice exam for a class. Closed-ended questions can be advantageous as they increase the standardization of data collection and ensure that the data collected will be in its intended format and easier to analyze. A downside to closed-ended questions is that you are forcing respondents into particular boxes. There may be individuals, for example, who don't strongly agree or strongly disagree with a particular question. If you are asking them to choose one or the other, it may not honestly represent their opinions or experiences. The type of closed-response question you ask could assist with decreasing the potential of this problem occurring. Table 6-1 provides information regarding and examples of various closed-choice question options within survey instruments from an example study about concussion in youth sports. Offering an option for "no response" or "not enough information provided" allows the individual to opt out from selecting a choice if they do not feel comfortable with what is provided. Additionally, inclusion of an "other" response with respondent options to fill in the blank may be advantageous.

   Closed-ended questions typically lend themselves to quantitative data analysis methods and may be useful when seeking information about frequency of occurrence in a population, averages of commonalities among participants, or statistical relationships among expected results and achieved results. This may include use of descriptive data or more complex statistical analyses procedures. Data visualization tools can also support observations of trends in closed-ended questions.

2. Open-ended questions: *Open-ended questions* in surveys are those for which the respondents are asked to answer orally or type a response to a given question. Choices are not provided, and thus, the collected data are truly unique to the respondent's own thoughts and ideas regarding the topic queried. These types of questions can provide rich and unique data points to enhance understanding of your area of study. As a person, I love open-ended questions. It is fascinating to hear what your respondents think about a given topic and it is interesting to look at both the similarities and differences among respondent perspectives. As a researcher, open-ended questions in surveys can feel like the most difficult thing in the world. There are a few reasons for this. The first is that I often find open-ended questions are interpreted differently by different people. When you don't provide a respondent with

choices, their brain has the ability to think about the question asked in its own unique way. You may receive answers that are completely different than what you intended the question to ask. You are subsequently left in a conundrum about how to analyze those responses. Speaking of analysis, a second potential hiccup to open-ended questions in surveys is that they must be analyzed qualitatively. In fact, surveys have been recommended as a tool for conducting qualitative studies (Braun et al., 2021). Qualitative research is amazing and I, quite frankly, wish we had a lot more of it in our field. However, qualitative methods take a great deal of time and care during the analysis phase. If you are looking for a survey to lend itself primarily to the quantitative world, open-ended questions might not be for you. I encourage you to include these in your surveys but also caution you to consider what type of information you are hoping to gain and what the data will be used for prior to beginning. Qualitative data analyses will be discussed in a subsequent chapter of this book. If you choose to incorporate open-ended questions into your survey research methods, you will want to be sure to review qualitative analysis methods.

## Participant Recruitment and Sampling

Prior to initiating a survey-based research study, a sampling plan (Montanari & Ranalli, 2005) must be developed. Knowing how many respondents you need for a survey study and understanding where and how to find those respondents can be quite difficult. A first potential step is to perform an a priori estimate of necessary sample size. A priori refers to decisions that are made before you begin the data collection efforts. If you look into the literature on research design, there are some that would suggest an adequate sample for a survey is 10% of the total population you intend to study. But in fact, I have seen numbers suggesting that up to 30% of the population of interest is needed for adequate sampling. That isn't so bad if your population of interest is the 40 graduate students in your clinical education cohort where a sample size somewhere between 4 to 12 respondents would suffice. Think about what that means, however, just for professionals in communication sciences and disorders at the lowest suggested sampling level. At the culmination of 2021, the American Speech-Language-Hearing Association reported having more than 223,000 members (2022). If we were to collect data from 10% of that population, we would need 22,300 responses. That makes me laugh (a lot) because I think the most responses I have obtained in a survey is just under 500—and those were college students who received compensation for participating. Now, of course not all American Speech-Language-Hearing Association members would be included in your target population. If you were to want information from speech-language pathologists who work

**Table 6-1**

# Closed-Ended Question Options in Survey Research

| QUESTION TYPE | DESCRIPTION | EXAMPLE QUESTION |
|---|---|---|
| Ranking | Respondents are provided with a list of options and asked to order, score, or compare the choices according to set criteria within the question | Rank the following service providers in order of importance when treating a youth sport-related concussion.<br><br>Pediatrician                                          1<br>Athletic trainer                                      2<br>Neurologist                                           3 |
| Agreement scales | Respondents select an option or move a dial to indicate their level of agreement or disagreement with presented information | It is important for parents to learn about preventing, identifying, and treating youth sport concussions.<br>☐ Strongly agree<br>☐ Agree<br>☐ Neither agree nor disagree<br>☐ Disagree<br>☐ Strongly disagree |
| Numerical scales | Respondents select an option that indicates a numerical value, such as frequency of occurrence or percentage of time | See table below |
| Adjective scales | Respondents select an option that may indicate their feelings or preferences relative to a presented item | How important do you think it is to learn more about how to prevent, identify, and treat youth sport concussions?<br>☐ Extremely important<br>☐ Very important<br>☐ Moderately important<br>☐ Slightly important<br>☐ Not at all important |

How much do you think playing sports has affected the following?

| | A Lot | Quite a Bit | A Little | Not at All |
|---|---|---|---|---|
| Learning about challenges/being a leader | | | | |
| Making new friends | | | | |
| Learning I had a lot in common with people from other backgrounds | | | | |
| I had good conversations with my parents/guardians because of sports | | | | |
| Improved academics (e.g., reading, writing, math) | | | | |

(continued)

### Table 6-1

## CLOSED-ENDED QUESTION OPTIONS IN SURVEY RESEARCH (CONTINUED)

| QUESTION TYPE | DESCRIPTION | EXAMPLE QUESTION |
|---|---|---|
| True-false or yes-no | Respondents select from a field of two to indicate a discrete choice of agreement or knowledge | Do you always wear your seat belt in the car?<br>☐ Yes<br>☐ No |
| Multiple choice | Respondents select from a field of greater than two choices to indicate a discrete choice of agreement or knowledge | Up to _____% of individuals experience long-term deficits following a concussion of mild head injury.<br>☐ 5%<br>☐ 15%<br>☐ 30%<br>☐ 50%<br>☐ I don't know |
| Select all | Respondents are provided the option of indicating more than one answer from a provided list of choices | What sports do you play?<br>☐ Football<br>☐ Track and field<br>☐ Basketball<br>☐ Gymnastics<br>☐ Baseball<br>☐ Swimming/diving<br>☐ Softball<br>☐ Rugby<br>☐ Soccer<br>☐ Field hockey |

in a school setting (about 97,000), the number would jump down to just under 10,000 responses needed. This still is not very feasible in my opinion. On the contrary, too few respondents (think back to the 4 to 12 number I referenced several sentences ago) may not be sufficient in reality to answer any clinical question in a meaningful way and will likely result in a survey study that is unsuitable for publication in the eyes of many journals. If this is the case, how do you figure out how many you need? There are many statistical methods available to help make an a priori sample size estimate. Resources exist to further explain these methods and the steps needed to complete them (e.g., Bartlett et al., 2001). To be honest, none of them are very user-friendly. My suggestion then, is to think critically about the goal of your study and the intended scope. In clinical education research, your intention may not be to study the whole of a population. Your aim might be to gain preliminary, but clinically meaningful information about a subset of the population whom you educate or who are involved in clinical education. Taking care to enhance your recruitment processes and understand/account for sampling biases will help to maximize your data collection efforts.

A potential advantage to survey research is that you may receive input from an unbiased sample of individuals. Depending on the type and extent of recruitment that you do, survey research may allow you to gain perspectives from individuals in diverse clinical settings, geographical locations, career stages, cultural and racial backgrounds, and professional experiences. In clinical education research, your participant recruitment and sampling may, however, be inherently biased regardless of your efforts. For example, if you are sampling only from your current university student cohort or from individuals who work as external supervisors for your university setting, you are gaining information from individuals that may already have positive or negative experiences with a situation or topic. Similarly, individuals who have strong feelings about a given topic in your survey may be more likely to respond than others. Let's take myofascial therapy as an example. If you are interested in learning about the importance of myofascial therapy in clinical education curriculum, you may receive more responses from rehabilitation professionals that feel strongly one way or another about the benefits of myofascial therapy. In physician assistant programs, there may be strong feelings regarding the minimum degree required to begin practicing or a change in title from physician assistant to physician associate. Psychologists might debate the relative value of the use of psychedelic drugs for the treatment of post-traumatic stress disorder. Thus, your sample is biased from the start. Although a different type of bias, the results you gain may still not be representative of the population.

One way to ensure that you are reducing participant bias is to recruit participants nationally. Reaching out to professional organizations who allow for recruitment on listservs or using approved social media platforms are methods to reach a wider audience from the commencement of your data collection phase. Another consideration is saturation in your recruitment (Guest et al., 2020). This concept will be particularly important in surveys that include open-ended questions that you might later analyze qualitatively. The term *saturation* refers to the point in data collection where no new information is discovered to be analyzed. In other words, it is the number of participants that are adequate to fully and accurately test your hypotheses. When you have reached a point of saturation, the research team may decide to stop data collection efforts and move fully to the analysis phase. This decision must be made based on the data you have and your team's own personal experiences and recommendations. Often utilized in qualitative research, this concept may be important when considering survey research methods and open-ended survey responses in particular. Even the best a priori sample size estimates may be inaccurate. Let me be clear—you should *never* review your data and make decisions on continuing or stopping data collection based on whether or not you have received the responses you expect or hope for. However, you may wish to review your data globally for variability of responses. High variability in responses may make it difficult for you to discern themes or trends in respondent perspectives. If high variability exists, you may have not yet reached data saturation and may require additional respondents prior to discontinuing data collection.

Another potential way to address respondent bias is to gather more information about the individuals completing your survey studies. Consider that you have initiated a survey and are recruiting individuals from across the country. You notice that your data are showing high levels of variability and large standard deviations. In such a case, it may be advantageous to break apart the data and discern response differences dependent on sample characteristics. For example, opinions regarding effectiveness of an educational program's diversity, equity, and inclusion policies from the perspective of former graduates may depend heavily on respondent characteristics, such as age, identified gender, racial and cultural backgrounds, time post-graduation, individual instructors or courses, and many more variables. By collecting this type of information about your respondents, stratification, that is, sorting people or data into groups and layers, of collected data is possible to enhance and clarify collected results.

# Data Evaluation and Interpretation in Survey Research

In the next section of this chapter, we will discuss additional options for inferential or descriptive statistical techniques that enhance interpretation of data findings within research across study types. Frequency distribution is the foundation for such techniques and an important first step in the statistical process. Specific to survey data analysis, frequency counts allow for further interpretation of data using measures of central tendency, measures of dispersion, and chi-square inferential statistics. We will discuss each of these briefly.

## Frequency Counts

Tallies or frequency counts refer to the number or percentage of people whose responses fit into a particular category. Similarly, frequency counts can relate to the number of times a phenomenon of interest or a particular response occurs within your data. Thus, frequency counts can be represented by percentages or absolute values. Frequency counts can elucidate information about three different measures of central tendency—or as you may remember them from middle school math: mean, median, and mode. The *mean* value within your data set is the average among all responses on a given question. Calculating mean is most useful when the response type is ordinal rather than categorical. For example, garnering the mean value of responses for a multiple-choice question with data represented as option 1, 2, 3, or 4 is not plausible. Although this seems straightforward, ensuring that you match an appropriate analysis plan with the type of data you have collected is key. When examining frequency of responses for a given item, *mode* reflects the most commonly occurring answer. The *median* value reflects the midpoint and may be useful when evaluating ranked data. Creating a frequency chart by aligning information from most to least occurrences is one manner of visually representing frequency data. In addition to measures of central tendency, measures of dispersion, such as standard deviation, range, and variance, may be necessary to gather to support inferential data analysis procedures.

*Chi-square* is a statistical test used to compare observed results in a given category to expected results in that category (Sharpe, 2015). Many readily available resources exist to support the understanding of the use of chi-square methods dependent on the statistical analysis program you are using (e.g., Microsoft Excel, R [The R Foundation], Statistical Package for Social Science [IBM]). The purpose of a chi-square test is to determine whether the observed patterns and relationships in the data are due to chance or due to your variable of interest (e.g., participant group, years of experience, pretest scores). Chi-square analyses should be used when comparing data from two categorical variables to illuminate a statistical value of significance (e.g., *p* value greater or less than .05). For example, following completion of a student survey, you might wonder if a statistically significant relationship exists between respondent ratings on your teacher evaluation and their achieved grade in their clinical practicum. This type of analysis can be particularly useful in survey research when attempting to evaluate relationships between responses on two independent questions or between participant demographic information and question responses.

# ADDITIONAL STATISTICAL METHODS

Here we are at the terrifying part that few people want to tackle—*statistics*. You don't have to be a mathematical wizard to conduct sound, evidence-based research in clinical education. When people ask me about the math involved in research, I often tell them, "I do statistics, not math." What I mean is that statistical analyses are methods available to evaluate outcomes for students and clients, interpret the impact of clinical decisions, and identify areas of growth and change in clinical education. These methods simply allow us to take the subjective out and allow the objective in. What they are *not* are convoluted math word problems about trains racing 54 mph down a track leaving the station at 3:15 p.m.

In both the single-subject and survey sections of this chapter, I provided you with information about some analysis methods that lend themselves specifically to those research types. These are not exhaustive lists. Additional statistical methods may be beneficial to answering your research questions and illuminating your findings. We will briefly discuss a few more statistical options next, but know that statistical methodologies are vast and far-reaching—many of them go beyond my professional expertise and require those with degrees in statistics and computational modeling to support implementation. The complexity of statistics can feel overwhelming and even I am continually learning new methods and enhancing my current knowledge. This doesn't happen overnight, so bear with me and be kind to yourself in this area of research. Again, phone a friend might be a great option here if you are feeling stuck. The scope of this chapter does not allow for us (thankfully) to fully highlight all statistical options. Rather my hope is to introduce you to concepts for later contemplation and in-depth learning.

## Data Visualization

If I said it once, I've said it 1,000 times, creating visual representations of your data may be the absolute most valuable research skill you can gain. This is no truer than in the world of single-subject and survey designs. Previously in this chapter we discussed visualizations of data and statistical methods for analysis and interpretation of results in both single-subject and survey design independently. However, data visualization is not limited to those procedures or benefits. In fact, graphically or visually representing outcomes for all research studies can be useful in observing patterns, identifying outliers, and making interpretations of outcomes. Creating visual representations of data is also highly influential when disseminating your research findings and creating a digestible representation of the numerical findings.

## Inferential Statistics

The traditional method that comes to mind when comparing data between two groups is the *t-test*. This type of inferential statistics involves calculating the average (mean) and standard deviation of a given dependent variable under more than one condition (e.g., group of respondents, experimental condition). The average data are then analyzed to determine whether a significant difference exists between the two points of comparison. In single-subject research, for example, the mean or average of an individual's performance on a dependent variable within each phase of the study can be calculated. Completion of a t-test can provide information about the presence or absence of a statistically significant difference between average performance within those phases to allow for interpretation of your intervention's effect. Presence of a *p* value less than .05 indicates significantly different behaviors between the intervention and non-intervention phases.

*Correlational data* allows you to evaluate the extent to which two pieces of data are related linearly or dependent on one another. What this means is that both variables of interest change at a rate consistent with one another. Although not commonly used to describe a cause-and-effect relationship, correlational data provides statistical insight into a general relation between two pieces of collected data. When completing these analyses, the correlation coefficient ranging from −1 to +1 is generated and describes the extent of the relationship between the two variables of interest. The closer the correlation coefficient is to 1, the stronger the relationship. Within these computations, statistical significance is again provided and indicated by a presented *p* value.

Another method for evaluating data using inferential statistics is the *analysis of variance*. These types of analysis are useful for dependent variables that are continuous in nature and allow you to determine whether there are statistical differences among the average data in three or more groups (Tabachnick & Fidell, 2007). First developed in 1918, this widely used measure can provide meaningful insight into data that is garnered from one individual across multiple variables (repeated measures) or between independent groups. Analysis of variance methodologies are useful when you are comparing more than two phases or more than two distinct pieces of information from your collected data.

# SUMMARY

Now that you've made it through this chapter without falling asleep (I hope), I know what you're thinking. "Where has she been all my life? I've finally found my research fairy godmother!" But seriously, my hope is that *somewhere* in this chapter you resonated with the information and considered the potential to transform your already amazing and innovative ideas into clinical education research. Is the information still a bit dry and boring? Probably. Let's be honest, it doesn't hurt my feelings. This brief introduction was intended to help you familiarize yourself with potential quantitative research methods that you could employ right away in your clinical education practices. I mentioned several times that aligning yourself with someone knowledgeable in research that you trust and have a positive, supportive relationship with will greatly increase the success of your team and your project. If you are going at it alone or are simply looking to dip your toe into the research pond, starting with single-subject and survey design methods are a great way to contribute meaningfully to your field of study while keeping your sanity. Good luck!

# REFERENCES

American Speech-Language-Hearing Association. (2022). *Annual demographic and employment data: 2021 member and affiliate profile.* https://www.asha.org/siteassets/surveys/2021-member-affiliate-profile.pdf

Bartlett, J. E., Kotrlik, J. W., & Higgins, C. C. (2001). Organizational research: Determining appropriate sample size in survey research appropriate sample size in survey research. *Information Technology, Learning, and Performance Journal, 19*(1), 43.

Braun, V., Clarke, V., Boulton, E., Davey, L., & McEvoy, C. (2021). The online survey as a qualitative research tool. *International Journal of Social Research Methodology, 24*(6), 641-654.

Busk, P. L., & Serlin, R. C. (1992). Meta-analysis for single case research. In T. R. Kratochwill & J. R. Levin (Eds.), *Single case research design and analysis* (pp. 197-198). Lawrence Erlbaum Associates.

Byiers, B. J., Reichle, J., & Symons, F. J. (2012). Single-subject experimental design for evidence-based practice. *American Journal of Speech-Language Pathology, 21*(4), 397-414.

Duckett, L. J. (2021). Quantitative research excellence: Study design and reliable and valid measurement of variables. *Journal of Human Lactation, 37*(3), 456-463.

Engel, R. J., & Schutt, R. K. (2016). *The practice of research in social work.* Sage Publications.

Fritz, C. O., Morris, P. E., & Richler, J. J. (2012). Effect size estimates: current use, calculations, and interpretation. *Journal of Experimental Psychology: General, 141*(1), 2.

Ginsberg, S. M., Friberg, J. C., & Visconti, C. (2012). *Scholarship of teaching and learning in speech-language pathology and audiology: Evidence-based education.* Plural Publishing, Inc.

Guest, G., Namey, E., & Chen, M. (2020). A simple method to assess and report thematic saturation in qualitative research. *PLoS ONE, 15*(5), e0232076.

Johnston, M. V., & Smith, R. O. (2010). Single subject designs: Current methodologies and future directions. *OTJR: Occupation, Participation and Health, 30*(1), 4-10.

Kraemer, K. L. (Ed.). (1991). *The information systems research challenge (vol. III) survey research methods.* Harvard University Graduate School of Business Administration.

Kratochwill, T. R., Hitchcock, J., Horner, R. H., Levin, J. R., Odom, S. L., Rindskopf, D. M., & Shadish, W. R. (2010). Single-case designs technical documentation. *What Works Clearinghouse.* https://files.eric.ed.gov/fulltext/ED510743.pdf

Lee, J. B., & Cherney, L. R. (2018). Tau-U: A quantitative approach for analysis of single-case experimental data in aphasia. *American Journal of Speech-Language Pathology, 27*(1S), 495-503.

Maggin, D., & Chafouleas, S. M. (2013). Introduction to the special series issues and advances of synthesizing single-case research. *Remedial and Special Education, 34*(1), 3-8.

Montanari, G. E., & Ranalli, M. G. (2005). Nonparametric methods in survey sampling. In *New developments in classification and data analysis* (pp. 203-210). Springer.

Parker, R. I., Vannest, K. J., & Davis, J. L. (2011a). Effect size in single-case research: A review of nine nonoverlap techniques. *Behavior Modification, 35*(4), 303-322.

Parker, R. I., Vannest, K. J., Davis, J. L., & Sauber, S. B. (2011b). Combining nonoverlap and trend for single-case research: Tau-U. *Behavior Therapy, 42*(2), 284-299.

Scruggs, T. E., Mastropieri, M. A., & Castro, G. (1987). The quantitative synthesis of single subject research: Methodology and validation. *Remedial and Special Education, 8*(2), 24-33.

Sharpe, D. (2015). Chi-square test is statistically significant: Now what? *Practical Assessment, Research, and Evaluation, 20*(1), 8.

Tabachnick, B. G., & Fidell, L. S. (2007). *Experimental designs using ANOVA.* Thomson/Brooks/Cole.

# Worksheet 6-1:
# Quantitative Research

How do you feel about quantitative research?

```
[                                                                    ]
```

Do you have people you could invite to your board of mentors who would be helpful with it?

```
[                                                                    ]
```

Do you have a research question in which you would like to measure something?
"Correlation between ..."
"Measure ..."
"Objective assessment ..."

```
[                                                                    ]
```

## Design Considerations

How might you design a quantitative study?

```
[                                                                    ]
```

What data collection methods might be used?

```
[                                                                    ]
```

Data analysis questions you have/want more information about/ask board of mentors about:

```
[                                                                    ]
```

# Qualitative Research Foundational Concepts

*Patrick R. Walden, PhD, CCC-SLP*

Research is an example of goal-directed behavior. Any goal-directed behavior will require a *belief* about one's context and what is *true* in that context, an idea of a *desired outcome*, an idea of *possible avenues* for achieving the desired outcome, and a way to determine if the avenue chosen was *successful* in achieving the outcome. One's belief about the research context and what is true is determined by one's philosophy of science. Having an idea of a desired outcome requires asking appropriate research questions, and ideas about possible avenues requires choosing appropriate research methods. Determining whether the chosen methods were successful requires appropriate analysis of the data using trustworthy means. This chapter introduces the reader to common qualitative philosophies and research methods as a means to provide the reader with a basis for beginning to conduct qualitative research. It is purposively introductory in its scope with the hopes that readers will experience initial success with basic qualitative methods and choose to delve deeper into qualitative philosophies and methods.

## PERSPECTIVES IN QUALITATIVE RESEARCH

In terms of one's belief about what is true, this chapter focuses on the *general interpretive perspective* in which the goal is to understand the meanings made by participants regarding a specific event or other phenomenon. Notice that the focus is on participant perceptions or ideas about something. Research participants' meanings about the world is what qualitative research is all about. Merriam and Grenier (2019) described this research as, "[being] mediated through the researcher as instrument, data analysis is inductive, and the outcome is descriptive" (p. 7). While there are a plethora of other approaches to qualitative research (see Patton [2014] for a detailed discussion of this diversity of approaches), Merriam and Grenier also stated, "The majority of qualitative research studies in education and other fields of practice fall under this [general interpretive] design and are labeled simply as 'a qualitative study'" (2019, p. 8). This basic yet widely used design is a solid starting place for those beginning to explore qualitative methodologies. All general mentions of "qualitative research" in

DeRuiter, M., & Ginsberg, S. M. (Eds.). *Clinician's Guide to Applying, Conducting, and Disseminating Clinical Education Research* (pp. 81-94).
© 2024 Taylor & Francis Group.

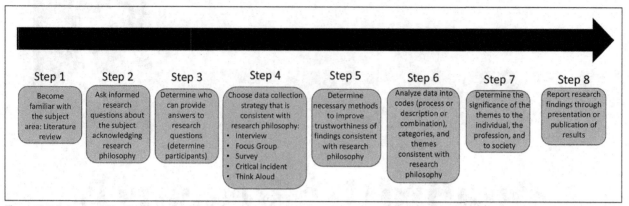

**Figure 7-1.** Sequence of qualitative research.

this chapter refer to this general interpretive perspective. The interested reader is encouraged to explore other research philosophies that support the conduct of qualitative research. Figure 7-1 provides an overview of the methods described in this chapter for quick reference.

# METHODS FOR ACHIEVING DESIRED OUTCOME: ASKING QUESTIONS AND GETTING THE DATA

Having a well-considered desired outcome for a research project helps focus the research question to include who the participants are, where they are (context), and what part of their experience is sought to be understood. If we view the world from a general interpretivist philosophy in which we view research participants' views and perspectives as sources of data, there are specific types of questions one would ask (an idea of a desired outcome) and specific ways to go about answering them (an idea of possible avenues for achieving the desired outcome). Qualitative research questions tend to begin with words like, "How does …," "Why does …," "What does …" They do not seek to count frequencies or determine statistical significance. Instead, they probe into the experienced realities of a population and are often contextually bound. For example, one might ask, "What do clinical fellows perceive as essential experiences during their initial face-to-face meetings with their clinical fellowship supervisor in urban rehabilitation centers?" This question seeks to gather information about participants' subjective experiences, sometimes referred to as "lived experiences," and the context for these experiences is explicitly stated.

The specific research questions asked determine the potential avenues for answering them. Some questions involve one person while others involve small or even large groups of people. Others seek to delve deeply into personal experiences/perceptions while others can be answered with less profound exploration. There are a range of methods to collect qualitative data and those data are almost always

texts or words in many health care–related fields, such as communication sciences and disorders. However, data might also be graphical if, for example, one is discussing augmentative and alternative communication systems. The most direct way to gather data from participants is to ask them to tell you what you want to know. This most often takes the form of an interview but can include holding a focus group and could also include portions of a survey. Sometimes you are interested in specific events in participants' lives and asking them to provide narrative accounts of these events is a source of data called a *critical incident*. Lastly, the clinical educator may be interested in learning about participants' thought processes and how or why they arrive at specific decisions about clinical situations. In this case, one may benefit from asking participants to perform think-aloud activities where the participant verbalizes their thought processes during an activity. Each of these is described next in terms of what types of questions lend themselves to these data collection methods, as well as how to conduct research using these methods.

## Interviews, Focus Groups, and Surveys

Interviews, focus groups, and surveys are grouped together here because they all share a common thread of asking individuals or groups of people a series of open-ended questions that will elicit data that will be analyzed to answer research questions. Interviews may be one-on-one or conducted with a small unit of people (e.g., a married couple, a caregiver and child). The role of the researcher in conducting interviews is typically to lead the conversations with the purpose of the research as a guide for structuring the conversations.

Focus groups are similar to interviews except the participants are made up of a "relatively homogeneous group," and they meet together to "reflect on the questions asked by the interviewer" (Dilshad & Latif, 2013, p. 192). The emphasis of the focus group participants' discussions is directly related to the research questions guiding the data collection, but the researcher's role is different for focus groups than that required of interview methods. Nyumba and colleagues (2018) described this difference as serving a role of "moderator" of the focus group participants' discussions rather than leading the conversation, as is common in interview scenarios. The researcher moderates the discussions in terms of facilitating the participants' interactions with one another. The data of interest in focus groups are the discussion and decisions reached by participants regarding the research topic (whether consensus is reached or participants provided divergent perspectives).

Surveys, in the sense used here, are similar to questionnaires. Survey designs that use a series of questions with prepopulated answer choices are not consistent with qualitative methodologies. Open-ended questions may, however, be added to these types of survey designs to elicit participant perspectives for which no prepopulated answer choices are possible or to further describe participant perspectives through additional data points that differ in nature. For example, if a survey focused on graduate student information-seeking behaviors when preparing therapy goals and asked the students to rate (on a scale) their level of agreement regarding the ample availability of the institution's resources, an open-ended follow-up question could be, "What is the process you use to access institutional resources when planning therapy goals?" One may find that a student reports via survey rating that they disagree that "ample resources are available" but then goes on to describe a process for accessing resources that suggests a lack of awareness of what is available or how to access any resources at all. In this example, only attending to the level of agreement regarding availability of institutional resources without the qualitative adjunct to this data point would have led to a very different conclusion regarding the appropriateness of the level of resources provided to the student. Instead, it could be the case that resources are ample, but the student does not know about their availability or is using an inefficient process of accessing them. As such, open-ended questions can serve as an illuminating data point in survey research.

Which of these methods one chooses will depend on the research question asked, as well as the overall purpose of the research (and available resources, such as recording equipment and space to hold groups of people). The types of research questions/purposes that may lend themselves to one method of data collection over another are described next.

## Asking Questions That Require Interviews, Focus Groups, or Surveys

Research questions that lend themselves to interview or focus group data collection methods are the types of questions that require a person to recount the unfolding of events or experiences or how they feel or perceive these events or experiences. These types of research questions often ask "how" or "why" questions, such as "How do school-based audiologists go about supervising students at multiple educational sites with long distances between sites?" This would require the researcher to ask clinical educators to describe their process (successful or not) for negotiating this situation. The purpose could be to look for common experiences covering the caseloads or to look for divergent or unique experiences in this situation. An interview, rather than a focus group, may be a better choice for this research question because the researcher will likely want to understand each individual participant's experience, providing a broader base for data analysis rather than seeking data through participant interactions with others.

For focus groups, questions that are best addressed through group interactions are applicable (Kamberelis & Dimitriadis, 2020; McLafferty, 2004). The questions may target ideas for which there is little previous research and for which a group discussion would likely provide the best understanding of the phenomenon. For example, Oommen and McCarthy (2015, p. 64) asked, "When addressing intervention for children with childhood apraxia of speech, among the areas of participation, literacy, language, and speech, how do experienced clinicians adopting the dual paradigm approach make decisions regarding the frequency and duration of therapy goals targeting natural speech?" This is a very specific topic about a specific client base and a specific approach. In addition, there are many parts to the research question. While these authors could have interviewed clinicians practicing in this area individually, they chose to conduct an online focus group in which the participants could interact with one another's perceptions while providing their own experiences. The synergy created from this relatively "homogenous" group provides a different set of data compared to individual interviews.

As stated earlier, open-ended questions in survey research serve to elicit participant perspectives for which no prepopulated answer choices are possible or to further describe participant perspectives through additional data points that differ in nature from the quantitatively measured survey items. For example, Swales and colleagues (2021) surveyed individuals in Australia with Parkinson's disease regarding communication and swallowing changes they experienced. One portion of the survey asked participants to indicate which symptoms they experienced from a prepopulated selection. As an additional section of the survey, open-ended questions were included, which prompted the survey respondents to recount their experiences with these symptoms and how they perceive them to be handicapping to their everyday life functions and activities. In this case, the purpose of including open-ended survey items was to further elucidate aspects of the "forced choice" parts of the survey. One note of interest about Swales and colleagues' (2021) study was that they used semi-structured interviews with people with Parkinson's disease as data to populate their survey items and the possible choices respondents could elect. While not discussed in this chapter, qualitative research is a viable means to develop theory that can later be tested through quantitative means.

## Collecting Interview, Focus Group, or Survey Data

Typically, interviews and focus groups are conducted face-to-face or online and are usually recorded for later analysis. Surveys are most often written in form, although surveys may also be collected through face-to-face interactions as well (e.g., political polling outside voting sites). In the allied health fields, the qualitative data will almost always be language that is somehow recorded. Transcripts of interviews and focus groups become the research data and are created to aid analysis and to facilitate multiple reviews of data with an audit trail (more on audit trails later in the chapter).

### Interview Guide

Research that is inductively analyzed (as in many qualitative methods) tends to require less preparation of the research instruments before data collection compared to experimental studies, and are instead more resource-intensive for the analysis and interpretation steps. That does not mean, however, that no planning occurs prior to conducting interviews or focus groups. Just as in any study, the relevant literature is reviewed prior to planning the study, but oftentimes, the subject matter of qualitative studies may be context-bound to the point that previous research findings may not apply, or it may be an un- or under-explored area where little-to-no research exists. In these cases, the research purpose and questions are the guiding principles for developing the research instruments. For interviews and focus groups, an interview guide is necessary to ensure that the interviews/focus groups cover all the areas of research interest but also to be sure that they focus only on issues germane to the research purpose.

Seidman (2019) described interview questions as being open-ended with the purpose of extending and delving more deeply into the participants' responses to the questions. Questions should be simple, easy to understand, and elicit descriptive responses. Researchers create interview guides to structure the interviews through listing these open-ended questions and their intended order of presentation. Roberts (2020) described interview guides as containing orienting questions, main questions, follow-up questions, and probes.

- *Orienting questions* familiarize the research participant to the interview process and may make the participant's role in the research process explicit. For example, an investigator may say, "Thank you for taking the time to talk to me about your experiences as a speech-language pathology clinical fellow. I am seeking a better understanding of your ideas, beliefs, and experiences as they relate to clinical supervision. Will you join me in this endeavor?" With this orienting question, the beginnings of rapport may be built, and the participant is asked to become an active part of the research process. The purpose behind the interview is also made clear for the participant.

- *Main questions* are broad questions meant to elicit respondent experiences and perspectives regarding the research focus (Roberts, 2020). These are the questions that deal directly with the participants' experiences and perceptions about the topic under study. For very loosely planned interviews meant to allow the participant to take more of a lead in where the interview goes, these may be the only type of questions prepared ahead of time. Although tempting to create a lengthy list, it is best practice to limit these questions to a small handful of questions written to elicit participant perspectives about your research. It is common that novice researchers develop too many questions, some only tangentially related to the study's purpose, and that the interviewer defaults to making sure all questions are asked in a checklist manner. It is much more important to focus your questions and *listen* to your participants' answers. The best interviews are really more like conversations than a strict question and answer format. Using the previous interview topic as an example, a possible main question could be, "How do you often feel after supervisory sessions with your clinical supervisor?"

- *Follow-up questions* are more micro-focused questions that tend to be more specific than main questions (Roberts, 2020). They can help ensure a deeper account of participant experiences and perceptions. They are designed to get more information. These are harder to plan because they typically flow from the content of the participant's responses. Asking for elaboration ("Tell me more") is a form of follow-up, as is nonverbal communication cues to continue (head nodding and investigator silence to indicate the participant should continue). Some main questions may lend themselves better to preplanned follow-up questions. Continuing the same clinical fellow supervision example from before, a follow-up question might be, "What do you think leads you to feel this way? What do you contribute and what do you think the supervisor contributes to this?" It is vital to remember that the primary task the interviewer is engaged in is listening. Having follow-up questions prepared does not require that they be presented if a participant has addressed them without direction. Asking a question the participant has already addressed is an assured way to cause the participant to disengage because they perceive they are not being heard. Active listening techniques that are common in clinical professional practices work well for qualitative research interviews as well. Your interviews will be more fruitful as a result of actively listening to your participants' responses as you go through the interview.

- *Probes* are a way to maintain the dialogue (or monologue; Roberts, 2020). They serve a social function for interviews and focus groups in that they can demonstrate that you heard what was said or to refocus a research participant. Using the clinical supervision example from before, one might say, "I hear what you are saying about your coworker's opinion of your clinical supervisor, but how do you feel that your perceptions are contributing to your participation in the supervisory process?" In this example, the researcher is reorienting the participant back toward salient aspects of the research vs. allowing the participant to go on tangentially. A probe could also be indications that the interviewer is listening (e.g., "mhmm"). Probes can also lead the research participant toward a desired response type, such as providing a moment-by-moment account of an event that is important for the research and will be probed in all interviews or focus group sessions. Probes such as, "Tell me exactly what happened, second-by-second, to the best of your ability to remember" can be common across interviews if the participant is not being specific. A list of potentially useful probes helps the interview or focus group move along in a smooth fashion.

The development of the interview guide is a crucial step in the research process. Questions must be crafted in a manner that elicits deep-level rather than surface-level responses. For example, a clinical educator-researcher may be interested in a group of students' responses to an interprofessional education event that included special education, physician assistant, psychology, and speech-language pathology students. The interview guide was populated with questions such as, "Tell me what you learned about working with special education students" and "Tell me what you learned about working with your peer speech-language pathology students." At first glance, these questions seem germane to the research interest, and they are open-ended. However, it is likely that the research participants will respond in a manner that only allows a list of "things" they feel they learned. This is an example of a surface-level finding (and one that could have been better measured through some type of mastery task aligned with the interprofessional education event's learning goals). A main question with two follow-up questions that are likely to elicit a deeper response may be, "Tell me about your interactions with your speech-language pathology peers. How did you go about using your knowledge during the event vs. relying on your peers' knowledge? Why do you think things unfolded that way?" The types of prompts used in qualitative research are one of the most important aspects to planning the research project no matter the data collection technique.

The best way to avoid surface-level questions is to pilot the interview guide. A co-researcher and one or two potential participants could serve as respondents and answer the questions on the interview guide. Based on the responses you receive, you can alter the interview questions as necessary. It is also possible to alter the interview guide during the research process if it becomes clear that the instrument is not providing the desired data (Rosenblatt & Wieling, 2018). Remember, you can only use these pilot data in your study if you have an approved institutional review board (IRB; see Chapter 9). Developing an interview guide that results in the data one desires is, however, best worked out before completing large numbers of interviews.

## Transcription of Interviews and Focus Groups

Transcription of interviews and focus group interactions have traditionally been seen as one way to become familiar with the research data because careful listening is required to accurately transcribe interviews and focus groups. McMullin (2021) suggested that researchers make note of the type of transcription being undertaken, as well as who is performing the transcription. Transcription is often done "verbatim," meaning that every word uttered is transcribed to record the event as accurately as possible. However, some researchers take written notes during data collection and then make transcriptions of the interactions from the handwritten notes. In addition, even for verbatim transcriptions, decisions regarding bracketed information (e.g., when someone laughs or if there is particular emotion in one's tone) must be made carefully. Deciding to add or ignore body language cues, paralinguistic features, and outward displays of emotion will alter the data itself. The decision to include (or not) these aspects should be considered in light of the research methodology being used.

Consideration of who transcribes the interviews and focus group interactions is equally important. Best practice is for the researcher to transcribe the interactions or to train anyone who is performing transcription so as not to alter the data in unintended ways. Remember, the interview or focus group transcript is the artifact to be analyzed in many cases. Transcripts made with errors or misrepresentations of quotes and events are not considered trustworthy and will taint analysis with altered data. While sometimes expensive, professional transcriptionists may be available and have experience transcribing audio data in an appropriate manner. For newer researchers, I highly recommend doing the transcription yourself (unless it is simply not possible).

While still not infallible, automatic transcription through artificial intelligence (AI) may be a viable means to reduce the high labor burden verbatim transcription requires (McMullin, 2021). Cloud-based AI that is free to use can transcribe interviews or focus groups, as well as allow for real-time collaboration of coding and other data analysis methods using shared, online documents. Most popular virtual meeting platforms provide real-time transcription of meetings, and these transcripts can be saved for analysis. For face-to-face encounters, audio recordings can be uploaded to popular video storage sites (e.g., YouTube) that use AI to create transcriptions for videos uploaded to the site. However, as Hopper and colleagues (2021) pointed out, use of such services should proceed with informed caution. There are potential privacy issues depending on where the data are stored and what the service does with the data (e.g., scan the data to supply relevant advertisements to the user). This is an issue that must be considered in the IRB application that serves to review research projects to ensure compliance with modern standards for protection of human research subjects. Confidentiality and privacy in research are necessary to protect research participants. Yet, use of these AI services may not pose any more risk to confidentiality and privacy than routine practices of everyday life. This type of risk-benefit analysis is an important conversation to have with colleagues and the IRB committee at the sponsoring institution. You can read more about IRB processes in Chapter 9 of this text.

# THE CRITICAL INCIDENT

Flanagan (1954) reported that the critical incident technique (CIT) began to be used as a means for psychologists to understand difficulties learning during aviation training in the 1940s. At its essence, CIT is the observation of human behavior to make inferences about vital aspects to successfully completing a task. It allows development of a set of critical requirements that have been observed across individuals who are successful at completing a given task. Through analysis of specific events across participants, the research can pull out common themes that seem critical to describing the event. Early on, CIT was used to provide guidance for developing a set of essential requirements for specific occupations, as well as for complex tasks/techniques. More recently, the technique has been used as a qualitative research method to better understand incidents from adverse sedation events in medicine (Coté et al., 2000), to developing a list of helpful and hindering clinical supervisory practices in athletic training (Curtis et al., 1998), to describing physicians' development from novice to proficient clinician (Sim et al., 1996).

For clinical educators, CIT holds promise in understanding what is critical for success in clinical practice in training students and new clinicians. Walden and Bryan (2011) explored clinical learning behaviors exhibited in medical settings and used CIT as one of several data collection methods. Through analysis of recounts of critical events that required on-the-job learning across several research participants, the authors used inductive processes to develop a process for using clinical learning behaviors in the workplace. To develop the process, analysis of multiple incidents across participants was required and those that seem common (critical) across the participants contributed to the model of learning in the workplace that was developed. For example, in Walden and Bryan's (2011) study, participants' reasons for engaging in learning behaviors at work were exemplified in the critical incident data and were compared to the reasons from other data collection methods (i.e., focus groups and individual interviews). This provided a level of "trustworthiness" to the reported reasons for engaging in learning at work because they were represented across many participants and from multiple data collection methods.

## Asking Questions That Require Critical Incidents

Research questions that suggest the use of analysis of the critical incident include those "that aim to acquire precise information on factors, events, behaviors, or experiences that result in satisfaction/dissatisfaction with care or that promote or detract from good quality delivery of care" (Viergever, 2019, p. 2). Research questions that seek to understand common components of a process may be fruitfully addressed using CIT. It is important to note that the critical components may be sought for successful processes (What is required for people to succeed?), as well as processes that turn out not to be successful (What is common among the processes used that turned out not to work?).

### Collecting Critical Incident Data

CIT data, like interview data, will be language-based. Most often, eliciting CIT data involves asking a participant to recount a time when an event of interest occurred, including all relevant details. For example, Walden and Bryan (2011) asked participants to, "[write] descriptive narratives describing a time or times when [you] encountered a clinical problem for which previous knowledge and experience were not useful in solving. Further, … [detail the] specific actions taken to address the problem and outcome(s) of these actions" (p. 382). In this example, the critical incident is meant to focus on a time when the participant's knowledge and skill were not successful in solving a clinical problem. As stated earlier, it is not necessary to collect data describing only "successful" events. There is much to learn about events that "go wrong" too.

Investigators can ask the research participants to orally recount the event, perhaps during an interview, or participants may be asked to write a narrative of the event and submit it to the researcher. It is this author's opinion that asking participants to write the event on their own and submit to the researcher is the preferred method to collect CIT data. If the event is not recent or is complex, it is likely that participants may forget key parts or require longer descriptions to include all relevant parts. Allowing the participant to craft the recount over time may increase the accuracy of the narrative. It is acknowledged, however, that CIT may be embedded into oral interviews and that having participants recount these events during the interview will reduce the amount of time required for their participation in the research. For recent events or events that are less complex, oral narratives of past events may not affect accuracy of the recount itself. Also, some participants may not be adept at written language and prefer or need an option to provide oral narration rather than written.

## Think-Aloud Method

The *think-aloud method* allows for inference regarding "what information is concentrated on and how information is structured during problem-solving task(s)" (Fonteyn et al., 1993, p. 430). At its essence, think-aloud is a process of data collection that asks participants to make their thoughts explicit (say them out loud) while they are performing a task or immediately after (Eccles & Arsal, 2017). For clinical educators, this method of data collection can access what is traditionally invisible to the researcher: the participant's thought process.

There is a range of research that has used this method. For example, Welsh and colleagues (2018) explored the thought processes of elite professional snooker players as they practiced alone (snooker is similar to billiards or "pool"). Along pedagogical lines, Nelms and Segura-Totten (2019) used think-aloud to compare how faculty engage with a research article vs. how novice students engage with the article. As can be seen, think-aloud allows thought processes to be made explicit and documented for analysis. The interested reader is urged to consult Ginsberg and colleagues (2012) for a think-aloud application directly related to clinical education.

### Asking Questions That Require Think-Aloud Tasks

The types of research questions that lend themselves to think-aloud include those questions that seek to explicate an internal thought process. Clinical educators may ask, "How do new student clinicians know when they are administering standardized tests with fidelity?" Another possible question is, "How do students successfully apply speech science knowledge to interpret acoustic data?" Any question that seeks to make explicit a participant's thought process may be addressed using think-aloud. As with the CIT method, the research question does not have to be posed in the positive. Think-aloud may be used to answer research questions about participants' thought processes when they are wrong, too.

---

> ## Box 7-1: Sample Script to Elicit Think-Aloud Data
>
> I am going to ask you to think aloud as you work through the test. Let me explain what I mean by "think aloud." It means that I would like you to tell me everything you think about as you work through each test question. You will do this one test question at a time. When I say tell me everything, I really mean every thought you have from the moment you read the problem to the end when you have a solution or even if you don't have a solution. Please don't worry about planning how to say things or clarifying your thoughts. What I really want is to hear your thoughts constantly as you try to solve the problem—uninterrupted and unedited. Sometimes you may need time to think quietly through something—if so, this is okay, but please tell me what you thought through as soon as possible after you're finished. I realize it can feel awkward to think aloud but try to imagine you are alone in the room. If you become silent for too long, I will say "keep talking" to remind you to think aloud … Let us now practice thinking aloud with two practice problems presented on your paper. What is the fifth letter after C? Now, please tell me everything you think about as you solve it (Wolcott & Lobczowski, 2021, p. 4).

### Collecting Think-Aloud Data

To collect think-aloud data, the researcher will ask the participant to perform a task and to "narrate" their thought process during completion of the task. It is also possible to ask the participant to recount their thought process immediately after completing a task if the task is relatively short and not overly complex. When the researcher is in doubt about task complexity, it is safer to favor during-task narration of the thought process. Wolcott and Lobczowski (2021) created an example script for eliciting think-aloud data, included in Box 7-1.

As can be seen in the example, the participant is asked to verbalize everything that they think while they are completing the task. This verbalization of thought is recorded and transcribed for later analysis. The same principles of transcription described for interviews and focus groups apply to think-aloud as well. It is key to be sure anyone who transcribes the recordings is trained to be as accurate as possible (and not take liberties with the transcription). It is also key to report what kind of transcription was made (e.g., verbatim). As the transcript is the artifact to be analyzed, its accuracy is vital to the success of the research.

# Did the Methods Achieve the Desired Outcome? Analyzing the Data in a Trustworthy Fashion

Analyzing qualitative data requires making sense and interpreting the texts that were transcribed through the chosen data collection method. Qualitative data analysis can take many forms and be simple or extremely complicated. The type of analysis a researcher undertakes will be informed by the research philosophy used to plan the study and collect the data. This chapter presents novice qualitative researchers with a general interpretivist approach, and consistent with that tactic, thematic analysis will be described as a means to analyze qualitative data. It should be acknowledged that there is no set of prescribed analytical methods for qualitative data and there are several possibilities for analysis even within the same research philosophies. It is not possible to cover qualitative data analysis in detail in one chapter. Indeed, entire texts have been written on this subject (e.g., see Miles and colleagues [2018] and Saldaña [2021] for detailed treatment of coding and qualitative analysis). Instead, a combination of approaches from Maxwell (2013) and Saldaña (2020) are combined here and described as thematic analysis. Both Saldaña's description of coding and Maxwell's process for collapsing codes into themes are trustworthy approaches to meaningful analysis of qualitative data.

## Thematic Analysis

Thematic analysis is a process that entails careful reading of the transcript and assigning pieces of language (can be a single word, short phrases, whole sentences, or whole paragraphs) some type of label. The type of label (code) assigned is based on the level of interpretation desired (more on this later). Codes are reviewed and grouped based on their similarities and renamed or "categorized" to better describe this similarity. These new categories are reflected upon to look for connections and meanings regarding the research questions and result in themes that illuminate the phenomenon explored. The themes are interpreted to report what has been learned about the research topic. As Thorne (2020) stated, reporting a list of codes, categories, or themes is not the end game of qualitative research. Instead, the interpretation of the themes is necessary "… to show us that there was some purpose in your having done so [divided up the transcripts into codes and themes] and to guide us into the new level of understanding that can be arrived at on the basis of an auditable explanation of the forays you have made into these different options for compartmentalizing, sorting, and interpreting data" (p. 2).

## How to Code and Develop Themes

A code is a stand-in for a larger piece of text. Its function is to represent meaning extracted from the text snippet. While there are many ways to code transcripts, this chapter will include process coding and descriptive coding. *Process coding* uses gerunds (a noun that is derived from a verb and ends in -*ing*) to exemplify the meaning of a piece of text while *descriptive coding* uses general nouns to describe the meaning text (Saldaña, 2020). A coder may use one type of coding to initially code the transcript and add other types of codes as necessary upon further reading and analysis of the transcript. The goal is to find the coding type that best fits the meaning of the text. There is no rule as to which types of codes should be used or if they can be used interchangeably. Again, the goal is to represent meaning, not fit a grammatical category.

For example, Walden and Bryan (2011) collected qualitative data from medical speech-language pathologists regarding their motivations for engaging in clinical learning behaviors at work. One participant responded with, "I am finding there is a lot of work politics … involved with this change [an organizational structure change] and although I speak to my colleagues, I need to be aware of what I say to others and how things are construed" (p. 385). Coding this piece of text would require that the coder know the context of this statement, including references to other events. In this case, the participant had been describing a recent change in the health care organization, including clinical processes and leadership roles. The participant was describing why they were engaging in learning in the workplace when they made this statement. Knowing this, a process code may be "treading lightly" or even "being cautious." A descriptive code might be "heedfulness." Different coders will certainly use different words for the codes themselves, but the meanings should be similar. Also, a code may be more than a word. In the present example, further analysis of the complete interview across multiple participants (and multiple data collection methods) indicated that the health care organization itself creates a need for employees to engage in clinical learning behaviors. As can be seen by this example, a single code is a minute piece of data and must be further analyzed to find meaning in the larger pool of data. A single code can, and should, be applied as often as necessary (as long as it adequately represents the piece of text). New codes are added as needed. All codes are carried over into the analysis of new transcripts and reused or added to as required to represent meaning of the text snippets. Coding of transcripts is an iterative process. It is added to (and subtracted from if necessary) to best represent the participant's experiences and perceptions.

Novice qualitative researchers often have misgivings about coding initially. Despite formal training in qualitative research methods, some new researchers will feel that the process is subjective and can vary from study to study.

These concerns are not surprising because they are accurate. Coding is subjective. Every coder sees the transcript through their own life lens, including experiences similar to those reported by participants, as well as experiences far afield of those reported. The key is that the coder makes a concerted effort to be aware of their own biases and experiences while coding. Taking the participant's perspective can help pull their meaning from the text. The coder must try to always be cognizant that they may be putting their own meanings on the participant's words. It is likely impossible to be completely free of bias when coding. However, there are ways to improve the trustworthiness of qualitative findings and those methods are described later in the chapter. For now, it is important to acknowledge that a true novice to qualitative research methods may not feel confident in their ability to code. The secret is that no one ever did when they first started, and coding is something that requires practice using transcripts meaningful to the coder. Divergent codes resulting from examples divorced of their context are often hard to reconcile among researchers.

Once transcripts have been coded, the codes themselves can be collapsed into *categories* (Saldaña, 2020) and then into *themes* (Maxwell, 2013). *Categories* are groups of codes that are similar in some way. The goal is to combine codes that share something in common, thus reducing the amount of data. A category can be one word or several words as long as it is descriptive of all the codes that fall under it. The category can take the name of a single code if the name is particularly demonstrative of the group's meaning. Also, a category could be made up of a single code if the code is different enough from the others to warrant its own category. The point is not to force codes into categories but to examine the codes and look for patterns in meaning. Similar meanings can be grouped and categorized together.

### Themes

A *theme* is an even higher level of classification. The theme is often what directly answers the research questions. Themes are developed by considering the categories and further combining similar categories as they relate to the research questions. Again, it is not necessary to force combinations of categories into a single theme. Instead, they should inductively "arise" from the analysis in as naturalistic a way as possible. The connections should be apparent through careful consideration.

In Walden and Bryan's (2011) study mentioned in the previous coding example, analysis of the transcripts yielded many different codes regarding motivations for learning in the workplace. Codes were collapsed into categories that included reasons internal to the person (e.g., lack of graduate training) and external to the person (e.g., unique presentation of communication disorder). They also included preclinical practice (e.g., during graduate training) and during novice and advanced clinical practice. Further examination of the categories led to one theme regarding motivation to engage in clinical learning behaviors. Specifically, the medically based speech-language pathologists engaged in informal learning at work to meet their patient's clinical needs, to meet their own personal learning needs, and to meet the needs of the health care organization.

As can be seen, individual codes were combined into more informative categories that then led to themes apparent across the participants. The analysis moved from specific units (codes) through more descriptive commonalities (categories) to a general description of the phenomenon of interest (theme). Analyzing codes and categories to develop themes may be helped by the use of reflective memos (Saldaña, 2021). Reflective memos are written accounts of the researcher's thought process regarding the data. They are similar to a diary or journal detailing the development of the analysis. They are usually dated and deal with the researcher's interpretation of codes and categories to make sense of the data. Initial ideas about themes are recorded in the memos to document the process of how themes emerge from the data. This makes the analytic process explicit and documents it for later audit as a means to demonstrate the trustworthiness of the findings. Use of memos or journals is also where the true implications of the findings may be explored. Moving a bit deeper in reporting of the research findings will require consideration of the findings as they relate back to the context of the participants, the field of study (e.g., the professional context), and the world at large. Only reporting the themes without tying them to a level of significance for the person, the profession, and/or society is an incomplete account of the research findings.

Lastly, reporting the themes that emerged from the research requires that individual quotes be used as "proof" or "demonstration" to the research consumer that the themes are supported by participant accounts. Themes should be reflections of participant experiences and perceptions as reported. If a researcher is having difficulty finding quotes that are apparent exemplars of the reported theme, there is likely an issue with analysis. The informed consumer would be wise to consider the quotes provided to support the emergence of reported themes and evaluate whether the quotes provide unambiguous support for the theme. If not, the trustworthiness of the findings should be questioned.

## Demonstrating the Trustworthiness of Qualitative Findings

Demonstration of rigor is an important aspect to qualitative research. Yet, there are no unanimously agreed upon set of rules for ensuring the quality of qualitative research. Entire texts have been published addressing the quality of qualitative research (see Seale [1999] for an excellent example). While positivistic approaches to research have a long history of ways to demonstrate validity and reliability of quantitative findings, the very mention of the concepts of "validity" and "reliability" can spark debate among various schools of thought regarding qualitative research methods (Bogdan & Biklen, 2007).

The term *trustworthiness* is generally accepted across qualitative traditions and its meaning refers to demonstration of the rigor with which the research was conducted. Demonstrating trustworthiness allows the consumer of the research a baseline of certainty that the findings reported are at least somewhat close to the participant realities analyzed. While no universal agreement regarding how to best demonstrate trustworthiness exists, a researcher can confidently use one or a combination of approaches to demonstrate rigor as long as the methods are consistent with the research philosophy from which the research project was designed. It should be noted that some qualitative traditions tend to require fewer of these methods to demonstrate rigor while others require several attempts to improve the trustworthiness of the findings. As this text is geared toward the clinical professions, it is recommended that qualitative research finding trustworthiness be considered carefully and a more conservative approach be employed (i.e., use more methods to demonstrate more rigor). Although some researchers' interpretations of qualitative research methodologies would refute this conservative approach, the reality of the state of research in some fields is far from fully accepting of qualitative approaches while some are more accepting of it. Also many researchers were trained solely in the positivistic tradition and lack a full understanding of what rigor is demanded according to different philosophical traditions. Luckily, the clinical fields are continually developing and ever more open to alternative ontologies and epistemologies, especially as they relate to understanding clinician and client perspectives in evidence-based practice. In that spirit, what follows is an explanation of common methods for ensuring the quality in qualitative research findings.

## Triangulation

Of all the methods for improving the trustworthiness of qualitative research findings, in this author's opinion, triangulation is the most important if the research seeks to explore commonalities in perceptions or experience. *Triangulation* is the use of more than one source of data in the interpretation of research data. Although the word "triangulation" suggests three sources of data, there is no rule that says it must be three. It can be two or 10. It all depends on the research study being undertaken.

Using more than one source of data in interpreting research data can take two forms. The first is that the research uses multiple methods of data collection. For example, the Walden and Bryan (2011) article often referred to in this chapter employed individual interviews, a focus group,

and collection of critical incidents. Each method collected data from different participants. When analyzing the data, codes and categories from all three methods were used to develop themes, and only themes with support from all three data collection methods were reported. This allowed the researchers to demonstrate a high level of commonality among the participant experiences, as they were able to show that they arose from three different types of data collection methods used with different participants. This is often referred to as the "groundedness" of the data, which depicts how often or how deeply a theme shows up in the data itself (more on groundedness later).

The second form of triangulation is using multiple sources of data within the same data collection method. Rather than collecting data in three different ways, the researcher can look for multiple instances of a code or category across participants or within the same participant's transcript. The purpose with this type of triangulation is to demonstrate that a theme was not developed from a single, one-off comment or recount of an event. Instead, it shows up multiple times in the data and is, thus, more "grounded." Some examples directly relevant to clinical education include triangulating clinical educator perspectives, student clinician perspectives, and/or client perspectives to look for common ideas.

It is not necessary to adhere to the level of theme representativeness (groundedness) reported by Walden and Bryan (2011). Themes that are exemplified frequently in the data can be reported without requiring that they emerge from every source of triangulation or from every participant in a single data source. The quotes used to support the reported themes can also strengthen the trustworthiness of findings that are not as frequently cited in the data itself, as long as they strongly exemplify the theme. Quotes that strongly support a theme are evidence that what is being reported is actually what occurred.

The purpose of the research will guide the researcher in determining whether triangulation is warranted or not. For instance, research purposes that seek to explore outliers or uncommon phenomenon may not benefit from triangulation of data. The very essence of the outlier may be diminished by requiring multiple sources of data.

## Coder Agreement

A common way to demonstrate that the codes and categories are representative of the data is to provide coder agreement percentage. To calculate the coder agreement, two or more individuals code the same transcript(s) separately and then come together and share their codes. The percent agreement includes how often the coders came to the same conclusion regarding a text snippet. This is done for the whole transcript or multiple transcripts. It is important to note that the code itself does not have to be the same word for both coders. If the meaning is the same, it may be counted as agreement. For disagreements, it is common that the researchers discuss the divergent codes and come to consensus regarding which code (or new code) best represents the data.

## Auditing

An audit trail is a group of documents or electronic files that may be reviewed by outside or other researchers and that describe the analytic process used to derive the research findings. It is a way to demonstrate that the research is rigorous (Carcary, 2020). Auditing does not require that the researcher change their research methods in any way. It only requires that all steps used in the research process (from initiation to development of findings) be documented in some way. This may include the audio recordings of interviews or focus groups, any transcripts that resulted from the data collection methods, any other correspondence with research participants (e.g., emails or notes regarding phone conversations), researcher journals or memos, or electronic versions of analysis (e.g., files used in electronic analysis of data).

Auditing is usually done after completion of the research; however, there is no reason that the efficient researcher could not include an external auditor as part of the research from the outset. This could potentially avoid realizing that more rigor could have been applied to a study only after it is complete. An external auditor should be well versed in qualitative research traditions and methods. The auditor should also indicate that they have the time required to dedicate to review of the often large amounts of qualitative data that result from this type of research.

## Reflexivity

Researcher reflexivity is a method to increase trustworthiness of qualitative research findings by explicitly attempting to identify and address researcher bias. At its essence, researcher reflexivity can be accomplished through researcher journaling or including reflection on the researcher's perspectives during writing of research memos. The purpose is for the researcher to reflect deeply on all aspects of the project in an attempt to identify their own perspectives and experiences related to the research. Further, these perspectives and experiences are used to look for "holes" in the analysis or "bias" toward particular interpretations of data. The researcher will, through reflection, attempt to remove their biases if possible. Researcher reflexivity is a means for the researcher to increase awareness about other possible interpretations of data that may be missed due to one's own experience.

## Member Checking

Member checking is a powerful yet simple way to improve the trustworthiness of the research findings. Member checking can take several forms, depending on the level of participant involvement desired. Member checking is accomplished by asking research participants to review research data and indicate if it exemplifies their experiences. For example, transcripts of interviews may be reviewed to verify that what is transcribed is what the research participant actually said (and actually meant). For further involvement, themes that emerged from the data analysis can be presented to the participants to determine whether they are consistent with what the participant provided and/or their perceptions and experiences. Last, research participants may be asked if the individual, professional, and societal implications of research findings reported include their perspective or if they are divorced from the participant's views or experiences.

Member checking is one of the most impactful ways to demonstrate that what is being reported is actually what research participants experienced. It allows broader participation in the research process beyond the principal investigator and a professional research team. Member checking is an avenue to assure the research consumer that, yes, what is reported is in line with the participants' realities and perceptions. That is the entire point of qualitative research after all.

## Using the Right Tools for the Right Job

Despite focusing largely only on an interpretivist research paradigm in this chapter, a lot of different research methods were explored, and a researcher may choose several of them even within one study. There is a much larger qualitative world than is described in this chapter. The large number of methodological possibilities can be both distracting and confusing for the novice researcher. While it was recommended at the beginning of the chapter to let the research philosophy dictate the research methods, it is not that simple in practice. Even within the same qualitative tradition, there are numerous methodological decisions to be made: What are viable data sources? Who are the best research participants? What counts as data? What type of coding scheme should I use? How involved should the research participants be? How many "quality" methods do I need to include to ensure rigor in the research? These are just a few considerations, and these types of questions can be overwhelming.

As mentioned earlier in the chapter, the allied health fields have historically leaned quantitative. In fact, they lean so far in that direction, they could tip over. The qualitative researcher in these fields should keep the overall profession (and its research proclivities) in mind when planning and conducting qualitative research. Some qualitative researchers would express displeasure in this sentiment and that is worthy of consideration. Qualitative research paradigms have their own traditions of methods and levels of rigor. There is no need to compare these paradigms to the positivist/quantitative research paradigms that are the norm in the sciences for most of modern history. Since neither approach can be philosophically refuted, they are both equally as important and useful to society. This is all true. However, the clinical educator delving into qualitative research methods should understand that some (e.g., communication sciences and disorders) fields are, for the most part, biased toward a more quantitative approach. This is certainly not out of malice, but more so familiarity. The vast majority of training programs in communication sciences and disorders focus almost solely on quantitative research. As such, the vast majority of researchers in the fields conduct research from this point of view. Fields such as physician assistants and pharmacology demonstrate a more balanced appreciation of the value of both quantitative and qualitative studies. Bias may also arise from external agencies that fund research grants (e.g., governmental grants), which skew very heavily toward quantitative research projects when grants are funded. So, understanding who will be judging the quality of qualitative research, as well as consuming it, is an important step for planning and conducting it. The purpose of research is to create knowledge that is in some way useful. As such, choosing qualitative research methods that are recognizable for those trained in the quantitative traditions may improve the dissemination of your qualitative research.

Choosing the "right" tools for your project involves examination of plans to (1) conduct a literature review, (2) ask research questions, (3) plan data collection and analysis methods, and (4) interpret research results in light of the underlying research philosophy. Simply choosing several methods to improve the trustworthiness of the research findings does not guarantee rigor. Instead, methods should be chosen purposely for their potential to add rigor and their consistency with the research philosophy and the research purpose.

This chapter provided an introduction to qualitative research methods from a general interpretivist perspective. It provided a general outline regarding potential sources of data and how to generally analyze the data. It is this author's hope that clinical educators will find this information useful and empower them to ask deeper questions about teaching, learning, and clinical supervision. We have much to learn about clinical training processes, and qualitative research methods may open doors that have been locked by a strict adherence to quantitative methodologies. Giving both approaches to research equally long shrift will lead to a more well-rounded and informative literature base from which to train future professionals.

# REFERENCES

Bogdan, R. C., & Biklen, S. K. (2007). *Qualitative research for education: An introduction to theories and methods* (5th ed.). Pearson.

Carcary, M. (2020). The research audit trail: Methodological guidance for application in practice. *Electronic Journal of Business Research Methods, 18*(2), 166-177.

Coté, C. J., Notterman, D. A., Karl, H. W., Weinberg, J. A., & McCloskey, C. (2000). Adverse sedation events in pediatrics: A critical incident analysis of contributing factors. *Pediatrics, 105*(4 Pt 1), 805-814. https://doi.org/10.1542/peds.105.4.805

Curtis, N., Helion, J. G., & Domsohn, M. (1998). Student athletic trainer perceptions of clinical supervisor behaviors: a critical incident study. *Journal of Athletic Training, 33*(3), 249-253. https://www.ncbi.nlm.nih.gov/pubmed/16558519

Dilshad, R. M., & Latif, M. I. (2013). Focus group interview as a tool for qualitative research: An analysis. *Pakistan Journal of Social Sciences (PJSS), 33*(1), 191-198.

Eccles, D. W., & Arsal, G. (2017). The think aloud method: What is it and how do I use it? *Qualitative Research in Sport, Exercise and Health, 9*(4), 514-531. https://doi.org/10.1080/2159676X.2017.1331501

Flanagan, J. C. (1954). The critical incident technique. *Psychological Bulletin, 51*(4), 327-358. https://doi.org/10.1037/h0061470

Fonteyn, M. E., Kuipers, B., & Grobe, S. J. (1993). A description of think aloud method and protocol analysis. *Qualitative Health Research, 3*(4), 430-441. https://doi.org/10.1177/104973239300300403

Ginsberg, S. M., Friberg, J. C., & Visconti, C. F. (2012). *Scholarship of teaching and learning in speech-language pathology and audiology: Evidence-based education.* Plural Publishing.

Hopper, T., Fu, H., Sanford, K., & Hinkel, T. A. (2021). YouTube for transcribing and Google Drive for collaborative coding: Cost-effective tools for collecting and analyzing interview data. *The Qualitative Report: Fort Lauderdale, 26*(3), 861-873. https://doi.org/10.46743/2160-3715/2021.4639

Kamberelis, G., & Dimitriadis, G. (2020). Focus group research: Retrospect and prospect. In P. Leavy (Ed.), *The Oxford handbook of qualitative research* (pp. 479-516). Oxford University Press. https://doi.org/10.1093/oxfordhb/9780190847388.013.24

Maxwell, J. A. (2013). *Qualitative research design: An interactive approach* (3rd ed.). SAGE Publications, Inc.

McLafferty, I. (2004). Focus group interviews as a data collecting strategy. *Journal of Advanced Nursing, 48*(2), 187-194. https://doi.org/10.1111/j.1365-2648.2004.03186.x

McMullin, C. (2021). Transcription and qualitative methods: Implications for third sector research. *Voluntas: International Journal of Voluntary and Nonprofit Organizations*, 1-14. https://doi.org/10.1007/s11266-021-00400-3

Merriam, S. B., & Grenier, R. S. (2019). Introduction to qualitative research. In S. B. Merriam & R. S. Grenier (Eds.), *Qualitative research in practice: Examples for discussion and analysis* (2nd ed., pp. 3-18). Jossey-Bass.

Miles, M. B., Michael Huberman, A., & Saldaña, J. (2018). *Qualitative data analysis: A methods sourcebook.* SAGE Publications.

Nelms, A. A., & Segura-Totten, M. (2019). Expert–novice comparison reveals pedagogical implications for students' analysis of primary literature. *CBE—Life Sciences Education, 18*(4), ar56. https://doi.org/10.1187/cbe.18-05-0077

Nyumba, T. O., Wilson, K., Derrick, C. J., & Mukherjee, N. (2018). The use of focus group discussion methodology: Insights from two decades of application in conservation. *Methods in Ecology and Evolution/British Ecological Society, 9*(1), 20-32. https://doi.org/10.1111/2041-210x.12860

Oommen, E. R., & McCarthy, J. W. (2015). Simultaneous natural speech and AAC interventions for children with childhood apraxia of speech: Lessons from a speech-language pathologist focus group. *Augmentative and Alternative Communication, 31*(1), 63-76. https://doi.org/10.3109/0743 4618.2014.1001520

Patton, M. Q. (2014). *Qualitative research & evaluation methods: Integrating theory and practice.* SAGE Publications.

Roberts, R. E. (2020). Qualitative interview questions: Guidance for novice researchers. *Qualitative Report, 25*(9).

Rosenblatt, P. C., & Wieling, E. (2018). Thematic and phenomenological analysis in research on intimate relationships. In *How qualitative data analysis happens* (pp. 50-63). Routledge.

Saldaña, J. (2020). Qualitative data analysis. In P. Leavy (Ed.), *The Oxford handbook of qualitative research* (2nd ed.). The Oxford University Press. https://doi.org/10.1093/oxfordhb/9780190847388.013.33

Saldaña, J. (2021). *The coding manual for qualitative researchers.* SAGE Publications.

Seale, C. (1999). *The quality of qualitative research.* SAGE Publications.

Seidman, I. (2019). *Interviewing as qualitative research: A guide for researchers in education and the social sciences.* Teachers College Press. https://play.google.com/store/books/details?id=OkmeDwAAQBAJ

Sim, M. G., Kamien, M., & Diamond, M. R. (1996). From novice to proficient general practitioner: A critical incident study. *Australian Family Physician, 25*(9 Suppl 2), S59-S64. https://www.ncbi.nlm.nih.gov/pubmed/8854408

Swales, M., Theodoros, D., Hill, A. J., & Russell, T. (2021). Communication and swallowing changes, everyday impacts and access to speech-language pathology services for people with Parkinson's disease: An Australian survey. *International Journal of Speech-Language Pathology, 23*(1), 70-82. https://doi.org/10.1080/17549507.2020.1739332

Thorne, S. (2020). Beyond theming: Making qualitative studies matter. *Nursing Inquiry, 27*(1), e12343. https://doi.org/10.1111/nin.12343

Viergever, R. F. (2019). The critical incident technique: Method or methodology? *Qualitative Health Research, 29*(7), 1065-1079. https://doi.org/10.1177/1049732318813112

Walden, P. R., & Bryan, V. C. (2011). Speech-language pathologists' informal learning in healthcare settings: Behaviours and motivations. *International Journal of Speech-Language Pathology, 13*(4), 378-388. https://doi.org/10.3109/1754950 7.2011.578659

Welsh, J. C., Dewhurst, S. A., & Perry, J. L. (2018). Thinking aloud: An exploration of cognitions in professional snooker. *Psychology of Sport and Exercise, 36*, 197-208. https://doi.org/10.1016/j.psychsport.2018.03.003

Wolcott, M. D., & Lobczowski, N. G. (2021). Using cognitive interviews and think-aloud protocols to understand thought processes. *Currents in Pharmacy Teaching & Learning, 13*(2), 181-188. https://doi.org/10.1016/j.cptl.2020.09.005

# Worksheet 7-1:
# Qualitative Research

How do you feel about qualitative research?

Do you have people you could invite to your board of mentors who would be helpful with it?

Do you have a research question that focuses on participant perceptions, experiences, or ideas about something?
    "How does …"
    "Why does …"
    "What does …"

## Design Considerations

How might you design a qualitative study?

What data collection methods might be used?

Data analysis questions you have/want more information about/ask board of mentors about:

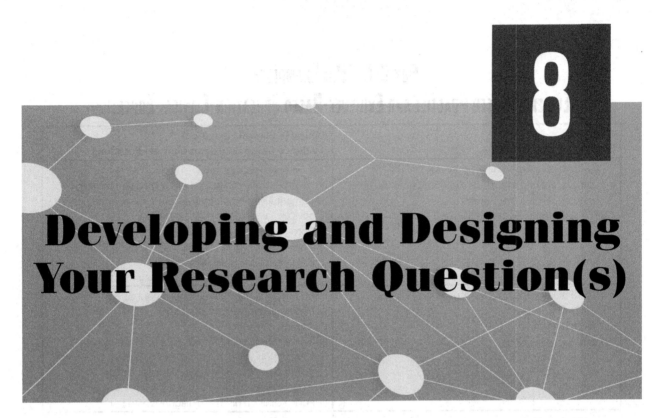

# Developing and Designing Your Research Question(s)

*Sarah M. Ginsberg, EdD, CCC-SLP, F-ASHA*
*and Jordan Dann, MA, CCC-SLP*

The co-authors for this chapter are both speech-language pathology professionals but from different backgrounds and bring different perspectives to this process. Sarah spent 12 years as a clinician but is now a university professor who has been conducting scholarship of teaching and learning (SoTL) research for about 20 years and has worked with dozens of master-level and doctoral students to help them develop their own research. Jordan is a community-based clinician working in a school with elementary and middle school children who experience a variety of speech and language delays. He was also a graduate student who completed his own research project in the form of a master's thesis. Sarah was his thesis chair. We have worked together before and felt that developing a new clinical education research question and pulling back the curtain into the process of working together, could give you insights into not only how to help your own research evolve but could illustrate how community partnerships, described by Lizbeth H. Finestack in Chapter 5, might unfold. The processes as described here are not intended to be prescriptive and followed step-by-step but rather to illustrate the way the process might look and feel.

## PICO Questions

Let's begin with the process for how you develop your searches for evidence-based practice (EBP) literature to address a clinical problem. One of the most common frameworks that has been utilized by clinicians in a wide variety of clinical settings to shape questions and facilitate a literature search is known as a PICO question (American Speech-Language-Hearing Association, n.d.; Hutcheson, 2017; Oregon Health & Science University, 2022). The reason that we are starting with this framework is because it might be familiar to you from your education and from your clinical work. In this framework each letter stands for an aspect of the clinical question:

P: Patient, problem, or population
I: Intervention
C: Comparison/control
O: Outcome

The PICO question gives us a structure to search the literature for information that will inform us of our best options for EBP with our clients. We begin by considering the patient or problem that we are faced with and the

DeRuiter, M., & Ginsberg, S. M. (Eds.). *Clinician's Guide to Applying,*
*Conducting, and Disseminating Clinical Education Research* (pp. 95-110).

## Box 8-1: PICO Examples—
## Evidence-Based Practice and Evidence-Based Education-Clinical Education

| Clinical (Evidence-Based Practice) | Clinical [+ Clinical Education] (Evidence-Based Education-Clinical Education ) |
|---|---|
| P: Pt. with apraxia; inpt. rehab<br>I: Augmentative and alternative communication device<br>C: Motor sequencing practice<br>O: Pt. independent ordering in restaurant | P: Pt. with apraxia; inpt. rehab<br>[+ new speech-language pathology graduate student]<br>I: Augmentative and alternative communication device<br>[+ novice clinician needs to learn device]<br>C: Motor sequencing practice<br>[+ novice clinician low confidence with motor skill knowledge]<br>O: Pt. independent ordering coffee<br>[+ novice clinician independent working with pt.] |
| P: Pt. with pulmonary congestion; urgent care<br>I: Diagnostic imaging<br>C: Auscultation alone<br>O: Pt. diagnosed correctly | P: Pt. with pulmonary congestion; urgent care<br>[+ nurse practitioner grad student]<br>I: Diagnostic imaging<br>[+ novice clinician confirm accuracy of reading image]<br>C: Auscultation alone<br>[+ novice clinician confirm accuracy of findings]<br>O: Pt. diagnosed correctly<br>[+ novice clinician discusses diagnosis with pt.] |
| P: Pt. complaint of fatigue; outpt. clinic<br>I: Order labs<br>C: Referral to other service<br>O: Pt. fatigue managed | P: Pt. complaint of fatigue; outpt clinic<br>[+ med student]<br>I: Order labs<br>[+ novice clinician ID what labs should be ordered]<br>C: Referral to other service<br>[+ novice clinician ID what services might be helpful]<br>O: Pt. fatigue managed<br>[+ novice clinician explains treatment options to pt.] |

characteristics of that group. We might be seeking information about a client of a particular age with a developmental disorder, for example. Narrowing down who the person is that we are trying to help or the characteristics of the problem we are trying to solve will help us begin to search the literature. We then need to look at what intervention we are considering for the evaluation or treatment of that disorder. In order to consider options for evaluation or treatment, we then will need to search for alternative approaches for the client. What other techniques have been tried? If the first or most common option is not appropriate or acceptable for some reason, what is a reasonable option that has the potential to yield a good result? Finally, what is the outcome that the client and you are seeking? Does your client want to have improved independence or be able to function in specific settings? Where is your novice clinician in the process? By considering the PICO elements, you will be able to search for literature that is relevant to your clinical practice, your clinical educator role, and the challenge that you might be facing.

In clinical practice, we may have used the PICO framework when we were faced with a problem. For example, I (SMG) have a client that is typical of clients on my caseload; however, when I use the approach that I would most often use with this group, I meet with a lack of success. Perhaps my clinical judgment has misled me, perhaps my client is atypical in a way that I didn't recognize, or perhaps they are simply not motivated to use the approach that I am recommending. If I am baffled, I have a clinical problem that will send me in search of an alternative intervention. In this case, it is often our first instinct to reach out to our colleagues who may have more clinical experience with the particular disorder if we have someone in our professional community that we think can be helpful. While this is valuable, consulting the literature is also informative and ensures that we are identifying evaluation or treatment approaches that are indeed evidence-based to help us solve problems.

## WHAT ARE YOU THINKING ABOUT?

When confronted with clinical problems, we can rely on the PICO framework and the EBP literature to guide us in determining an appropriate course of action to evaluate or treat a client in the best EBP manner possible. But what happens when we have a problem that is based on our role as clinical educator? In the early stages of SoTL, Randy Bass (1999) posed a critical question about teaching: "What's the problem?" (p. 1). He noted that, in science, when we come upon a problem that needs to be solved, it's a good thing—it indicates an opportunity for research. However, when we come upon a teaching problem that needs to be solved, it can be seen as a problem to hide. We might think that the problem reflects poorly on us as the educator, rather than on the context, the learner, or the content. It seems the culture of higher education does not always support or promote the open discussion of challenging learning situations, leading us to feel it must be a shortcoming on our part rather than a really complicated client or student or both. Most of us who have been clinical educators for any length of time have had similar problems or questions that go through our heads when working with students. We might wonder how they arrived at a conclusion based on the information they were given. We question their interpretation of a research article in its application to a particular client. We consider what causes them to react to feedback in a particular manner.

These are the problems that keep us up at night wondering what is happening, what we should do, or if an idea we have might work to solve the problem. When you consider the evidence-based education-clinical education (EBE-CE) model, there are a great number of questions that may arise from any of the intersections between the practice of EBP clinical work, the practice of EBE with students, and your role as a clinical educator. The most important thing to start with is to ask yourself what you find yourself wondering about. As our colleague Dr. Jennifer C. Friberg (2018, p. 3) would ask, what are the "problems?," what are the "opportunities?," and what are the "wonderments?" you might have around problems associated with clinical education. Based on the work of Hutchings (2000), Friberg describes "problems" as those questions that arise when things are not going the way you would want or expect. "Opportunities" may be considered in a more favorable view in that they may be related to what you think would work or are excited about trying in clinical education. "Wonderments" reflect more of the creative potential to integrate or add a component that is conceived of by the clinical educator. These are good problems to have because they represent an opportunity for learning from the literature and the potential to study the situation.

As you reflect on the challenges that might be keeping you awake in the middle of the night, consider what the broad topic is and what terms might be that are associated with it. In order to move from "I have a problem" to finding a solution, we must develop a strategy for searching the literature. We discussed in Chapter 3 that in finding the research, you might need to get creative with your search terms, and depending on the database you are using, search broadly and use a variety of synonyms. At this stage in your thinking, you will want to read as much as you can about your topic. Your goal is to learn as much as you can not only about the topic you are interested in but also what has been studied about it already, how they studied it, and what they learned. You might find inspiration for your study design in reading about others' designs in their research. The next sections will guide you through that process.

## DEVELOPING YOUR QUESTION

When discussing how we think of the process of developing and shaping a research question, both authors simultaneously described it as a process of *distillation**. We say this because, like distilling Scotch, the process of conducting research often starts with large amounts of an unrefined, raw material (literature) that after a series of steps eventually matures and develops into a focused, finished product (research study) that is satisfying to the researcher and the readers of that research, much like the process of distilling a fine Scotch. Our graphic represents the parallel processes between distilling and research in Figure 8-1.

(*Please note that we are not advocating or condoning consumption of alcohol, merely using the production process as an analogy for "distilling" your interests into a final product that you will be happy with.)

### Gather Grain/Read Widely

In the first step of developing your clinical education research question, you will need to start with raw ingredients. You have questions about a clinical education situation that might focus on the student's learning, the client's progress, or the intersection of your role in each. You will want to start by learning broadly as much as you can about the issue. This will require some initial exploration in the literature. You might consider returning to textbooks from your student days to refresh your knowledge about what you were taught (if that is relevant). If it is a topic that you were never taught about, you might start with broad sources, such as Google Scholar, PubMed, or your professional organization's sources for peer-reviewed literature. At this point, you are gathering enough grains of information to begin shaping your current knowledge about the topic. Finding meta-analysis articles, systematic reviews, and literature reviews can be very helpful at this stage if they are available. At this point, you will want to read broadly, learning everything you can about the topic. "Read, read, and then

| | Gather Grain | Cook | Ferment | Distill | Age | Bottle |
|---|---|---|---|---|---|---|
| **Scotch** | Grain is gathered from a field and dried. | Water is added to the grain, heated, and cooked, becoming *wort*. | The wort is put in a new container with yeast. As it is heated, the yeast converts to sugar, which produces alcohol. | The mixture is then put into a still that, when heated, causes the alcohol to evaporate up into tubes. When it cools, it becomes pure alcohol. | The alcohol is put into an oak cask. The cask (and whatever it might have held in it previously) imparts flavors into the Scotch over time as it is allowed to age. | Once the Scotch has been aged and taken on the desired characteristics of the cask, it is bottled so that it can be enjoyed. |
| **Research** | Read widely | Find the gap | Identify emerging questions | Assess feasibility of questions | Refine question and design study | Conduct research |

**Figure 8-1.** Distilling analogy for research development.

read some more" (University of Michigan Dearborn, 2022). Consider reading beyond your own field and look for content that may be useful in informing your thinking in related fields. Each of our disciplines may have conducted research with different populations for different purposes. As a speech-language pathology educator, I often find valuable SoTL work in the fields of nursing, psychology, and medicine. Reading the literature from other clinical professions and related fields may enlighten us and move our thinking forward.

A common question that arises as novice researchers are trying to gather as much information to begin this process as they need is how much is enough and when do you stop? I usually recommend that you read until you feel that you have a strong sense of what the current standing of the issues are. Read until you start reading articles that refer to the articles that you have already read. When you read a newer article and find that you have read most of the articles that appear in its literature review, there is a very good chance that you have adequate foundational knowledge to begin to move forward. There are a lot of data to keep track of in this search process: key concepts, theories, significant researchers, and areas that you have explored. Just like using a recipe book to keep track of your ingredients, you might want to use a journal or spreadsheet to keep track of

your materials and process. Sarah is old school—she uses a notebook for this, while Jordan is more prone to spreadsheets. However you approach it, try to develop your own system for keeping track of what you have done.

## Key Questions to Ask Yourself

What do you know? What do you know about your topic? What is the foundational knowledge related to it? What seems to be the current trend or direction for work in this area? Whose/what work seems to be referenced repeatedly?

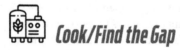 *Cook/Find the Gap*

Now that you have your raw ingredients of the literature gathered, it is time to add water and start the cooking process. As you read, you will probably start noticing key researchers who are writing about the topic that is of interest to you. You might discern patterns that become evident in what is being discussed or researched. As you are cooking down all your grain, infused with your new knowledge and perspective, you might begin to realize that while you know much more than you did to begin with, there are perhaps pieces of information missing. There is knowledge you are

# Box 8-2:
## Strategies for Finding the Research Gap

1. Look for trends in the focus of the research for the past 5 to 10 years. Some questions that might be useful to ask yourself come from Editage (Qureshi, 2019).
   a. "What is the significance of this research to my work or the broader field?
   b. How can this article help me formulate my research questions?
   c. Does the author's argument require more clarification?
   d. What issues or questions has the author not addressed?
   e. Is there a different perspective that I can consider?
   f. What other factors could have influenced the results?
   g. Are the methods or procedures used outdated or no longer considered valid in my field? Is there scope for me to test the findings using a more current approach?"
2. As you read the research, explore the discussion sections of the articles.
   a. What areas are identified as *future directions* for further research?
   b. What aspects of the research left unanswered questions?
   c. Are any of the study's results ambiguous? What could be clarified?
   d. What *limitations* of the study could be overcome with a new study?
   e. Are there participants for whom the results may be valuable but were not studied?
      i. Race, ethnicity, cultural, or linguistic backgrounds
      ii. Socioeconomic groups
      iii. Gender
      iv. Context (such as inpatient vs. home care or urban school vs. rural)
      v. Age of the client
   f. Are there different types or aspects of data that were not gathered that might be informative (quantitative, qualitative, mixed method)?
3. Talk with other people about your topic.
   a. What questions do they have?
   b. What have they read?
   c. How do they perceive the issue?
4. Keep a list as you read and talk to people.
   a. What questions do you have?
   b. What do you feel is missing?
   c. What do you want to know more about?

seeking but isn't present. At this stage, you are starting to identify what researchers often refer to as the *research gap*. Research gaps are the aspects of knowledge that have yet to be fully explored. This could be an aspect of the research that has only been recently conducted and so has not been addressed widely yet. It might be that there is research that tells you correlates of a behavior or condition (quantitative data), but none that has explored *why* the correlation exists (qualitative data). You might see that the research has been conducted on one group of individuals, such as English-speaking adults, but not on bilingual speakers, thus

a segment of the population has yet to be examined. Finding the gaps in the research is key to your progress. If you are new to this process, consider a few items that might be helpful to you as you sift through the grain and start cooking.

## Key Questions to Ask Yourself

What don't you know? What seems to be missing from the discussion? What aspects of knowledge haven't been explored yet? What contexts, groups, and perspectives are unexplored? Are there flaws or missing elements in current studies?

| Consensus | Sweet Spot | Controversy |
|---|---|---|
| • Well established views<br><br>• Facts widely accepted<br><br>• Little room for vastly different view<br><br>• *Nothing new here* | • Shared understanding but possible differences in applications, conditions<br><br>• Questions add to current understanding by exploring new perspectives<br><br>• *Much but not all is known* | • Inadequate agreement to foster valuable discussion<br><br>• Not enough information to agree or disagree on<br><br>• *Nothing known* |

**Figure 8-2.** Finding the research question sweet spot. (Adapted from Klopfer, L. [2022, February]. Selecting a topic. *Eastern Michigan Library Research Guides.* https://guides.emich.edu/c.php?g=567673&p=3916495)

## Ferment/Identify Emerging Questions

You are probably getting a sense of the direction that your cooked ingredients are going in at this stage, so it is time to let them ferment. It is time to see what happens as you consider what aspects of the research gap you identified from before you might want to address. If you have done a wide range of reading in the first step and then critically reflected on identifying the research gap in the second step, you likely now have more questions than answers. Identifying the research gap will give you a sense of next steps to consider, but it doesn't mean you are ready to conduct research just yet. Much like the liquid in our distillation process that is fermenting and maybe beginning to bubble, the ideas in your mind need some time to be processed, too. You can begin to develop emerging questions that arise from the gaps you are identifying. Look at your list of all the questions and consider how you might ask a question that could be answered by research you could conduct. Think of this as a brainstorming session. Your job at this point is not to determine which questions are the best questions, but just to generate a list of questions that both need to be answered and that you have an interest in answering.

After you have created a list of possible questions, you can begin to sort the questions into three categories as depicted in Figure 8-2 (Dunn, 2009 as cited in Klopfer, 2022). The first category of research questions are those questions where there is already consensus. You might have minor variations based on the knowledge, but if a finding has been accepted as fact for a long time in your field, it may not be worth your time to investigate further, depending on your skills and knowledge. Depending on your field, you may find that little clinical education research has been conducted. You may well find that you don't have much in the consensus category. As you review your list, you might find

that another set of questions is too controversial, too far out of the realm of current thinking, to make them possible to tackle. Research questions that represent controversy are seldom the place for initial research questions or first-time researchers. There may be a lack of enough consensus around them to even facilitate a productive dialogue within your discipline. They may be difficult to manage as you move them forward trying to receive funding, professional support, and get them published. The middle category is what Dunn (as cited in Klopfer, 2022) termed "the sweet spot" because it is the place where there is enough consensus to have a discussion but there is still an opportunity to explore differing views and perspectives. This is often a good place to position your early research efforts.

### Key Questions to Ask Yourself

Could I replicate a study but with a different group of people? Could I conduct a similar study but in a different context? We know how an outcome correlates with a condition or situation, so can we explore why? What happens if we change one variable from a previous study? If a behavior is demonstrated, can we determine how they arrived at the outcome?

## Distill/Assess Feasibility of Questions

As the focus of our questions start to take shape, we must then turn our attention to determining if the questions could feasibly be answered. Much like the liquid in the still, our questions are becoming less diluted, more focused on moving toward an end product. We often start with wonderful questions that for a variety of reasons we won't be able to answer. Here is a useful tip: Don't throw those questions away. Find a place to store them for the future. You never know when the opportunities you have will change and you might be able to reconsider them. We would recommend having someplace to store research questions, whether that is on paper or electronically. Sometimes collecting them all in one place not only gives you a chance to revisit them down the road when your situation may change (perhaps you applied for and received a grant that will pay for the materials you need!), but it also helps you develop a sense of your own thinking and curiosity about clinical education research over time. I also find that this list can be handy to call up when I'm talking with others (e.g., students, clinical educators, academic researchers) about the intersections of our interests if we are considering working together.

Alright, back to things to consider as you assess the feasibility of your research ideas. For you to be successful as a clinical educator researcher, you want to set yourself up for success. That means not undertaking a study that you cannot be successful with or complete. Starting with a question that cannot be answered is the surest way to find yourself frustrated and giving up. That is why this step is crucial. Undoubtedly, the vast majority of clinical educators reading this book do not have unlimited resources or support for conducting research. As the potential research questions run through your mind, consider what resources you might need to conduct your research. Below are some specific aspects of research and resources that you might want to consider.

## Scope of Question

In my (SMG) experience of working with many graduate students who want to conduct research for a thesis, they will often begin this stage by having very large-scale research ideas. In the case of a graduate student, they are likely to have multiple limitations on their ability to answer big-picture questions. I often tell them they have a great question, but because of the many limitations in resources (that we will discuss next), they are unlikely to complete their work. As complete work is always the goal, I help them consider the likelihood of being able to complete the work and narrow it down to something they can be successful with. Here are some examples of questions that start with a wide scope and can be narrowed down to something achievable.

## Time

Narrowing your scope will be the first step in considering if your study can realistically be conducted. The next, and perhaps most important consideration, is time. Many clinical educators find themselves squeezing this research into their already full days of working with clients, supervising students, and the many other tasks that eat up your time and attention, such as serving on committees. You likely do not have the luxury of allocated time for research. Of course, you may have nothing to lose by asking those you report to if there is any form of support, including a unit of time built

### Box 8-3:
### Narrowing the Scope of a Question

| Broad Scope | Narrower Scope |
| --- | --- |
| Format of feedback (oral vs. written) preferred by clinical educators in speech-language pathology | Format of feedback (oral vs. written) preferred by clinical educators in speech-language pathology in university clinics |
| Student perceptions of stress in nursing graduate programs | Student perceptions of stress for nursing graduate students in first semester clinical experiences |
| Are novice pharmacology clinicians afraid to deliver bad news to patients? | How does observation of a role model delivering critical patient education influence a novice clinician's confidence relaying drug information? |
| Is ultrasound training in physician assistant programs beneficial? | Does ultrasound training in physician assistant programs improve preceptor evaluations during the emergency medicine rotation? |

into your schedule for conducting this research. Depending upon the institution's priorities, they may say yes—as your mom might have said, "You don't know until you ask." Recognizing that time is a high value commodity for most clinicians and most facilities, we are going to assume that you have no fairy godmother granting you a block of time. In that case, you need to realistically consider how much time you have available in your life and how to design the research so it can be conducted in that time frame.

## Access to Resources

There are a number of resources that you should consider as you begin identifying potential research questions. If your first thought is *I don't have that* or *I'm not sure how to get that*, don't assume that you cannot get it. Start by noting that you would have to find a solution or mechanism by which you could gain the access you need. You never know when professionals in your community might have what you need and would be willing to partner with you or just support you in your efforts. This connects back to the ideas about building a research community/board of mentors that you read about in Chapter 5.

## Access to Participants

As researchers, we often come up with ideas about studies we could conduct if only we could get access to the right people. Ask yourself if you have the ability to access the database that you would need in order to get the data for analysis. Do you have a way to connect to the group of individuals whose perspective or data you want? Are you affiliated with an organization, or do you have the contacts to be able to find your way in and get the people you want to have participate in your study. For example, I might be interested in conducting a study about how doctoral students mentor new graduate student clinicians, but if I don't have access to doctoral students (because I am not affiliated with a doctoral program) who are doing this kind of clinical education, where will I find them? Doctoral students are busy people. If I don't have an in or a connection to them, I may not get enough to participate in my study to make it meaningful. I might be able to solve the problem by partnering with a colleague who does work with doctoral programs, but unless I find a way to access the target population that I want to study, my research may not be fruitful.

## Access to Literature

Be sure that you are confident in your ability to access the literature you will need to learn the foundational knowledge you need to develop your study. This might be as simple as learning how to access journals available through your professional association or your employer. It might be more complicated if your professional association journals are insufficient. You may need to rely on colleagues in settings who have library subscriptions for a wider range of journals. These colleagues may be university professors or clinical educators, but they may also be professionals who work in an organization that has library privileges (such as a larger health care system). Contact local library districts to see what databases they are able to access and contact local university libraries to see if they grant any access to people in the community. They may let you come in and read material, you just may not be able to access it online or sign material out. Also be sure to acquaint yourself with the mechanisms, such as a Google Scholar search, and broader search engines, such as WorldCat. See Chapter 4 for more information regarding searching the literature.

## Access to Instrumentation/Technology

You may find that in order to conduct your research, you need resources that will help you gather data. For example, if you want to conduct survey research, you will need to identify mechanisms for developing and sending out surveys. Similar to finding literature, you might start by finding out what your own employer has access to, as well as identifying any resources that your professional association offers. In addition to partnering with colleagues who have resources you need, explore what is available for free or very inexpensively. There are a number of websites that will allow you to create surveys free or at low cost. Explore your options using your web browser and look for the fine print regarding limitations. Perhaps while conducting your literature search, you came across a questionnaire that you think would be perfect for identifying students' perceptions of your topic. While the questionnaire might be copyrighted, a number of entities (including state and federal government websites) may be willing to grant you use of the questionnaire that you find on their website. Additionally, you would be amazed at how many researchers are willing to share tools that they have developed with fellow researchers. You may have to do a little sleuthing to find out who developed the form or questionnaire, and then figure out where they are now to find their email addresses, but in my experience, this is often easier than you might think and can be extremely helpful.

## Funding

While the scope of this workbook limits our ability to adequately address issues of funding, it is important to mention that there are sometimes funding options available that may be helpful to you in supporting your research efforts. Consider both internal (funds available from within your institution or organization) and external (funds available from sources that are not affiliated with your organization) opportunities. You may also want to investigate what, if any, financial resources are available from your professional organization. While large amounts of funding are often highly competitive and onerous to apply for, you might be surprised at how accessible smaller grants, particularly those designated for local communities, may be for you. If you are interested in pursuing funding to support your research, consider investigating options on the internet, talking to your employer, and also consulting your board of mentors (Chapter 5) for more help.

## *Collaborations*

Collaborations were addressed in Chapter 5 as the concept of building a research community/mentors was explored. However, we would be remiss if we did not mention here that finding others to work with can be invaluable to your research process. Collaborating with colleagues can have a myriad of benefits. Some of those benefits may include:

- Having a colleague to discuss and refine your ideas with
- Finding a colleague who has expertise in areas that are different from yours, and therefore, increases your potential effectiveness as a researcher

- Working with a person who has access to materials and resources you don't have
- Sharing the workload and time burden with another professional
- Holding each other accountable to complete work and move the project forward (Thanks, Jordan!)

### Key Questions to Ask Yourself

What type of information will I need to answer this question? Do I have access to the participants that I would like to study? What will the data that I collect look like? Can I access the technology/instrumentation that I need to conduct this research? How much time will this research realistically take to conduct, and can I do it? Will collaborating with another person to complete this work increase my likelihood of success?

 ## Age/Refine Question and Design Study

After mulling over the questions of feasibility regarding your research, you are probably getting closer to having a research question that can be answered. In this second-to-last step of the distillation process, we are going to put the finishing touches on your research question and study design, just as our Scotch is being refined by taking on some of the characteristics of the wood cask that it will sit in for a period of time. As we have begun to narrow the possibilities of how we will form our research question and design the study, we need to continue reflecting on the best options that are available to us. It is important to word the research question, which is often abbreviated "RQ" in research materials, in a clear and concise manner. There are a number of ways that you can think about developing your research question that will help you shape it in a way so as to be engaging, feasible, and valuable (George Mason University Writing Center, 2018; Nelson & Goffman, 2006; SUNY Empire State College, 2022). Here are some suggestions of characteristics to consider in writing your research question.

As you begin wording your question, thinking about what you want to know will help lead you to the wording of your question. Quantitative studies that seek correlation may begin with words that imply which is better, faster, or stronger, in some way, such as "Which method decreases time for assessment completion?" or "Does teaching EBP with a particular tool increase diagnostic accuracy in student clinicians?" Questions that seek understanding about a process or a phenomenon may ask about "how" and "why" questions to begin with. Chapters 6 and 7 will be useful for you to consider how you want to word the question. Your wording should suggest the nature of the research,

---

## Box 8-4: Writing a Research Question

☑ Specific: Your question should be very specific and say what you want to learn. The reader should be able to identify the focus of the study easily.
  ☒ Vague: Avoid questions that feel open to interpretation or are unclear.
☑ Focused: The study purpose is narrowed enough so that it can be answered easily.
  ☒ Overly narrow: Is it so specific that there will be little interest to a large segment of readers.
  ☒ Too broad: If the research question is written so broadly that it could be interpreted in a variety of ways or apply to a variety of people or contexts, it may not be effective in adding information to the literature.
☑ Concise: Write it directly to the point in as few words as feasible.
  ☒ Wordy: Try to edit it to be brief and reduce lengthy wording/phrasing in the question.
☑ Measurable/gatherable: Can you reasonably expect to collect the data that will be needed in order to answer your question?
  ☒ Immeasurable: Avoid questions that will require you to collect more than is possible given your resources, cannot be easily be gathered, or cannot be measured.
☑ Complex: The question is not answered with a clear "yes/no" but requires a deeper level of synthesis and analysis to develop new insights into the phenomenon being studied.
  ☒ Simplistic: If the question is worded in such a way that there is little room for debate and discussion, it will not add to the body of literature that helps us be an EBP and EBE-CE–guided field.

---

quantitative or qualitative, as well as what you are seeking to learn about. Research questions evolve over time. Consider how your thinking has evolved over the course of this distillation process and moved from questions that were on your mind as you engaged in clinical education to become more focused as you learn what is known and unknown about the topic. This evolution continues as you work to get the wording just right in this stage.

### Key Questions to Ask Yourself

Is my question specific? Is my question focused? Is my question worded concisely? Is my question answerable with measurable or gatherable data? Is my question complex in nature?

## Study Design

Once you have a reasonably clear research question developed, you must design the study in order to answer the question. Study design is "the set of methods and procedures used to collect and analyze data on variables specified in a particular research problem" (Ranganathan & Aggarwal, 2018, p. 184). We have already asked some questions related to accessibility and feasibility questions. Now you need to think about what data will be collected in order to answer your research question. Remember, the data you collect and analyze must answer the research question in order for your research to be of value. If you are looking for data from students, you will need to consider completing the institutional review board process, as described in Chapter 9. If this is your first time conducting clinical education research, we suggest that you begin with a method that feels the most approachable while still being able to answer your question. Consider the approaches that were discussed in Chapters 6 and 7. Which seems like a good fit for your inquiry? Will you be conducting an experimental design study in which you will manipulate independent variables? Will you be conducting an observational study where you try to understand the process of thinking or learning that underlies the phenomenon that you are investigating? While many would hold the randomized controlled trial up as the gold standard of experimental research, we must acknowledge in clinical education research that it is not likely to be feasible due to time, money, and a lack of ability to randomly assign participants to different groups. Instead, we should consider if we need to conduct an observational or an interventional type of study (Ranganathan & Aggarwal, 2018). Interventional studies are those where the researcher performs an intervention, perhaps giving the student clinician simulation experiences in addition to their clinical caseload, to see if the introduction of an independent variable (the simulation experience) changes a test score, which serves as the dependent variable, in comparison to students who do not receive the simulation-based education. You may be able to gather data over time that allows you to compare students who have differing learning experiences (from one semester to the next, for example).

Observational studies are those in which the researcher does not manipulate any variables and instead attempts to measure or observe a naturally occurring event or process in the educational or clinical setting. What is more likely to be feasible are observational studies in which you can collect data from student clinicians. One consideration in determining the feasibility of your study design may come from the literature that you have been working so hard to gather. As you reflect back on the research that brought you to this stage of the process, consider study designs that were implemented by previous researchers. If the study design has been used previously, it may signal to you that it can be done without too many hurdles and it may also increase the value of your work by making it comparable to the work that has been completed previously (Price, 2013).

### Key Questions to Ask Yourself

Do I want to manipulate the learning process or observe it as it naturally takes place? Do I want to study an individual, a small group, or a cohort? Do I want to compare one group to another?

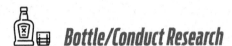 ### Bottle/Conduct Research

You may be thinking to yourself that this distillation process has taken an awfully long time and a lot of work, and we haven't even conducted a study yet. This is true of our Scotch, too—a lot of hours of labor have gone into getting the liquid ready to drink and making it be the best that it can be. The labor is worth it because the steps we have taken will increase the likelihood that our research will not only go smoothly but that the data we collect will answer our questions and our colleagues will appreciate it as much as that fine Scotch when we share it with them. Once you have refined your research question, you will proceed to the process of conducting the study. This is often the most gratifying step as all of your work from the previous weeks and months starts to pay off.

## CASE STUDY APPLICATION

Now that we have explored the various aspects of distilling and bottling a research question, let's apply this model to a case study, as depicted in Figure 8-3. The idea for this example came about as an exercise in thinking about the process of gathering information (Gather Grain) and developing and refining a question and study design (Distill). As this workbook seeks to encourage and empower clinical educators of all disciplines to begin research, the case study holds a broad scope. Naturally, when embarking on your own process, your specific practices will look different. Nonetheless, we felt it best to model the process.

### Gather Grain/Read Widely

To begin, I (JD) reflected on topics that pertain to clinical education in a relevant manner. Given the myriad of changes in the world, education, and subsequently, clinical education, I was curious about how "stress" as a phenomenon was understood in graduate school programs and how clinical educators could support the wellness of graduate students. From this meditation, my first "wonderments" surfaced: "How are clinical graduate programs encouraging healthy coping and stress reduction among students?" and "How are clinical educators supporting stress management among graduate clinicians?"

| | Gather Grain | Cook | Ferment | Distill | Age | Bottle |
|---|---|---|---|---|---|---|
| **Research** | Read widely | Find the gap | Identify emerging questions | Assess feasibility of questions | Refine question and design study | Conduct research |
| **Case Study**<br><br>How do clinical educators support the mental health of grad student clinicians? | Explored literature with curiosity, developed PICO document, identified relevant key word searches | Gathered work from key authors, correlated findings with other disciplines, identified shared concerns | How does a multi-modal approach to stress reduction influence graduate student clinician emotional resilience? | Curricula and resources, time, measurement protocols, funding | Direct mind-body instruction, self-reflection, yoga, SKY breathing work, control groups | |

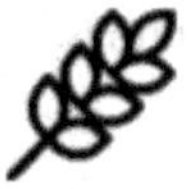

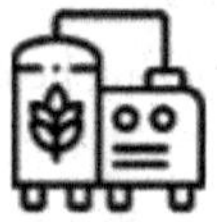

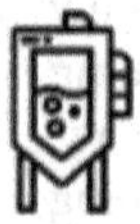

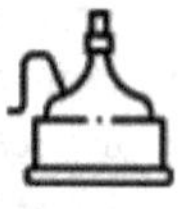

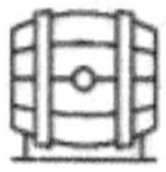

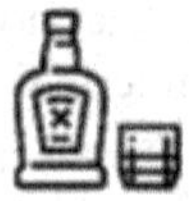

**Figure 8-3.** Distillation application—case study.

At this point, I got very curious and started exploring the literature. I began a list of key words, such as *mental health, graduate school*, and *stress*. After digging in, I found articles that resonated with me and my initial question, of which excited me. For example, Lieberman and colleagues (2018) aimed to survey the root causes of stress among speech-language pathology graduate students. I found other articles and university website postings that suggested a variety of ways graduate programs were helping their students manage stress. I kept notes in a hybrid document that used the PICO process to create space for me to ask questions, pull snippets of quotes, reference other articles, and expand my thoughts. This was vital for me because the information was becoming unwieldy. For example, in a study conducted by Seppälä and colleagues (2020), the SKY Campus Happiness program and the Foundations of Emotional Intelligence correlated to significant positive changes in mental health factors, such as reduction of depression, and an increase of positive affect and social connectedness, among others. My PICO notes for this entry included:

P—Participants: Undergraduate students on a medical track

I—Intervention: Three mental health programs (e.g., SKY Campus Happiness)

C—Comparison: Separate groups by intervention (i.e., Foundations of Emotional Intelligence, Mindfulness-Based Stress Reduction), compared to one control group

O—Outcome: Positive gains in mental health factors (e.g., stress reduction)

As a sub-bullet to this PICO entry, I also included the ponderings "what does SKY mean?," as well as notes about new terms I was learning, such as mindfulness-based stress reduction (MBSR). As an aside, I fell down a rather large "rabbit hole" regarding the SKY breathing technique (Sudarshan Kriya, which are various calm and rapid rhythmic breathing patterns), of which the SKY program utilizes (Zope & Zope, 2013). I say rabbit hole because I found more articles about that breathing technique in correlation to stress reduction, which led to more curiosities, such as "How might yogic breathing techniques benefit clinical graduate students?" After all, incorporating breathing techniques could be an inexpensive and effective way to promote coping strategies in clinical programs. Sarah helped pull me out of that rabbit hole with a well-timed suggestion. I spoke with Sarah early on in this process to express my findings and excitement. She was immediately reminded of recent research that directly pertained to my questions. Remember the board of mentors that was discussed in Chapter 5? That was happening in real time. Sarah, having much more experience with the research process, was able to see into my process and relate it to other relevant work. Sarah suggested that I review the work of Shah and Galantino (2019). This study anchored my wonderings into my field (speech-language pathology), and feathered out other aspects to investigate, such as didactic- and writing-based conflict management skill development; the study also incorporated articles that I was previously referencing, such as the work by Beck and colleagues (2015) that incorporated yoga. After exploring Sarah's suggestion, I found authors that were referenced in Shah and Galantino's article that produced literature that was very relevant to my wonderings (Box 8-5). This is a good example of locating the "sweet spot." I dug into the other articles by those authors and read up on their most recent research. In doing so, I also saw new authors reference that research (some websites have a handy "Where is this material being referenced?" section, so check them out!). I now felt like I entered a flow of research to which I was excited to contribute. You never know which colleague or practitioner will share an intersection with your question, so be open and share your curiosities with others.

> ## Box 8-5: Jordan's PICO Notes Regarding Shah and Galantino
>
> Sarah and I spoke recently, and I mentioned my interest in studying breath work with graduate students. She mentioned a study by Amee P. Shah and Mary Lou Galantino (2019) that I read for this search.
>
> - PICO Information:
>
>   P: Undergraduate students in communication sciences and disorders
>
>   I: During each class period, students engage in a worksheet-based empowerment curriculum, rating scales, mid- and end-of-semester reflection
>
>   C: No comparisons
>
>   O: Increased measures of self-esteem, emotional regulation, and communication competence
>
> - This article expands my understanding of thriving. The four domains of growth described seem very holistic.
> - I see article titles in the reference list that include "yoga," but no explicit practices were noted. However, there were three by Beck and colleagues that may be valuable to read next.

To manage the articles I found, I first reviewed them for relevance, then downloaded them using the name template "Lead Author. Year. Title." I saved the articles in folders by general category, such as "Nursing," "Undergraduate," and "Meditation," among others. I moved files around as new categories popped up. This helped me organize broad topics, which influenced my searching patterns. For example, the study by Vermeesch and colleagues (2017) titled, "Interventions to Reduce Perceived Stress Among Graduate Students: A Systematic Review With Implications for Evidence-Based Practice," became "Vermeesch.

2017. Interventions to Reduce Perceived Stress Among Graduate Students A Systematic Review With Implications for Evidence Based Practice." I saved that article in the "Nursing" folder, which allowed me to see correlations between differing health disciplines.

> ## Box 8-6: Jordan's PICO Notes Regarding Vermeesch and Colleagues
>
> - Article ("Interventions to Reduce Perceived Stress Among Graduate Students: A Systematic Review With Implications for Evidence-Based Practice") references breath work, Beck and colleagues' and Bond and colleagues' work, no SKY or breathing during class … more treatments. *What does this illuminate?*
>   - What does Bond and colleagues' work say? (need to read)
>   - What is "MBSR"?
>     - Mindfulness-based stress reduction!!
>   - Notes breath work in practice

As I noted before, I used my PICO notes to keep track of wonderments and new key words. I often found new topics to study in the middle of reviewing an article. After I finished exploring that particular vein for wondering, I reviewed the new key words and searched them. I also used my notes to highlight interesting studies that I found within the reference page of other articles, paying special attention to recurring authors. As I updated my notes, I highlighted new concepts and terms that various studies presented in their findings. A sampling of those terms included allied health, MBSR, embodied health, empowerment, emotional resilience, yoga, breathing, and reflection. My searches expanded to nursing, medical schools, and speech-language pathology programs.

 ## Cook/Find the Gap

After identifying key authors of interest and correlating their findings and suggestions with other pilot studies and systematic reviews, the "grain" began to "cook down," revealing *research gaps*. More specifically, current studies in medical schools, nursing programs, and speech-language pathology programs were all studying how to reduce stress within specific learning communities. I started to think about how different pieces of what has been tried could be combined, including new selections of participants and control groups. I saw direct instruction being paired with guided reflections that facilitated conversations. I saw community-building exercises increase camaraderie and emotional intelligence. I saw specific breathing practices referenced, along with yogic postures. Many of these studies shared correlations, but no two studies utilized the same coping mechanisms, data metrics, or participants. The literature from undergraduate premedical programs focused on understanding the neuroscience of stress reduction through the vehicle of breathing and body awareness. Speech-language pathology literature focused on modes of empowerment via writing and group dialogue within graduate programs, as well as yoga and mindfulness. Nursing literature produced systematic reviews of studies highlighting stress-reducing modalities within clinical programs. A possible intersection emerged from these findings and included elements of direct teaching, mindfulness, breathing, and guided practices/activities.

## Ferment/Identify Emerging Questions

At this stage, I have located a few studies that represent the core of my wonderings. These studies include:

1. "Building Emotional Intelligence for Student Success: A Pilot Study" (Shah & Galantino, 2019)

2. "Promoting Mental Health and Psychological Thriving in University Students: A Randomized Controlled Trial of Three Well-Being Interventions" (Seppälä et al., 2020)

3. "Interventions to Reduce Perceived Stress Among Graduate Students: A Systematic Review With Implications for Evidence-Based Practice" (Vermeesch et al., 2017)

4. "Embodied Health: The Effects of Mindbody Course for Medical Students" (Bond et al., 2013)

5. "Yoga as a Technique to Reduce Stress Experienced by CSD Graduate Students" (Beck et al., 2015)

Ultimately, new wonderments kept bubbling up. How do these various programs relate, and how can I contribute to this research? What methods of stress reduction in university programs produce the greatest impact? What is missing among these studies, such as the use of control groups or didactic teaching paired with guided practices? How can I combine the most impactful modalities into a new study, and what would that look like? What metrics did these studies use? Was there a principle or phenomenon at play vs. a specific and prescriptive method being uncovered (e.g., awareness of breath vs. Sudarsha Kriya breathing specifically, a select empowerment curriculum vs. writing and sharing about one's emotional resilience)? I allowed these bifurcating questions to grow and circle back onto one another, fermenting into a central question: What combination of stress-reducing modalities produce the greatest impact among graduate clinicians?

## Distill/Assess Feasibility of Questions

Now that I am closer to a research question, I need to consider the feasibility of the current question. For this, I will unpack how scope, timing, access to resources, and collaboration intersect my question. Regarding the scope and time of the question, I began my wonderings by seeking to understand how graduate clinicians can engage stress-reducing practices to enhance their learning process. It would be fabulous to create a longitudinal study, track students during their program, follow up with them after the program, and look at trends over time. A wonderful idea, right?! But I need to scale this back, something Sarah tells me often. (Thanks for helping maintain my sanity, Sarah!) I think a reasonable scope for this question is to look at how specific, manageable (we will define this) modes of stress-reducing practices (as informed by the literature) affect one or two cohorts of graduate clinicians over the course of one or two semesters. I don't want to interrupt the already packed course of study (much?) or add stress-inducing demands on clinical educators and graduate students (that would be counter-productive and ironic …). In fact, some of my core studies suggested beginning classes with a brief stress-reducing practice and adding one additional "task" for that week's requirements; this seems manageable. Regarding access to resources, I need to find graduate clinicians to engage in a study, locate the curricula and guides for stress reduction (or create it), and consider the metrics of which I will use to gather data. I also need to get clear on what the "data" actually is. I love the rating scales that many of the studies I found utilized, so I began to look into them with the hopes to use the same ones. For now, I am looking to simplify and use what was already created—plus, it allows for better comparison to previous studies. As one of my core researchers used her own published curricula, I plan to reach out to her as a collaborator and see if her material (and insight/encouragement) is accessible (e.g., affordable, easily implemented). The general idea here is to get really specific about the what and how of my study and put reasonable expectations around them to create a successful study design.

## Age/Refine Question and Design Study

At this point, my question is entering the age/refine phase. The goal of this phase is to build out the research process. I intentionally left my question broad enough to encompass a selection of different modalities, so now it's time to get specific. Additionally, many studies warned against the lack of control groups, so I am making sure that is accounted for in my upcoming study. As an aside, I wrote an initial draft of my study design, and in true Jordan fashion, the design grew into an overly complex, four-way design that would have required qualitative and statistical analysis. Thankfully, Sarah is well familiar with my rabbit hole–bounding, and she reminded me that crafting a more concise study would be most successful. I realized that I held the fallacious thought that the study needs to address *all* of the questions to close the research gap; this is, of course, not true—focusing on even one aspect of the research gap is valuable and meaningful. After some reflection and collaboration (Thanks, Sarah!), I decided to focus on combining two stress-reducing methods as one group and compare it to a control group. I thought through the research question using the principles previously outlined in this chapter (specific, focused, concise, measurable, complex):

- Research Question: How does a guided empowerment curriculum paired with rhythmic breathing exercises influence stress reduction among clinical graduate students?

As the research question suggests, I plan to study how the use of the empowerment curriculum (Shah & Galantino, 2019), in conjunction with specific breathing practices (Sudarshan Kriya), influence the reduction of stress among graduate clinicians. My study design includes two groups: one group who participates in both guided empowerment curriculum and breathing exercises, and one control group for comparison. I will plan for the first 10 to 15 minutes of a class to teach these practices, as well as some manageable homework to generalize the practices. I will collect data using the rating scales outlined in the study by Shah and Galantino, as well as use mid- and end-of-semester writing exercises. Both groups will use the rating scales and writing exercises, in efforts to compare findings. My study will focus on understanding the phenomenon of stress reduction and will be analyzed using the principles of qualitative analysis.

## Bottle/Conduct Research

Now that the research question is established and the study designed, I transition to implementing the study. This includes writing my proposal and research instruments. As well as getting institutional review board approval, gathering my participants, preparing my resources, and last but certainly not least—conducting the study. Wish me luck! Cheers!

## CONCLUSION

We made it! In this chapter, we unpacked the process of crafting a research question and designing a study. The method of distilling Scotch served as a working metaphor to understand this process. We discussed reading the academic literature widely (Gather Grain), finding a research gap (Cook), and identifying emerging questions (Ferment). We then assessed the feasibility of those questions (Distill) and refined the question and study design (Age). The final stage of the process is to conduct the study (Bottle). This journey was made specific using a case study in which an initial "wondering" was "distilled" into a research question and study design.

The authors sincerely hope that this exploration empowers you to get curious and find a path to formulating your own research study. As a practicing clinical expert, you hold a unique intersection, one filled with diverse personal experiences and insight. Your field, as well as adjacent fields, will benefit from your findings. Over time, our fields will grow more robust and connected because of the research you contribute. Future students will thrive, and their future clients will experience this positive impact, as well. So, observe the growing grain of your personal "wonderments," harvest that wheat, and get to cooking and distilling. We look forward to reading your research!

## REFERENCES

American Speech-Language-Hearing Association. (n.d.). *Step 1: Frame your clinical question [PICO elements]*. https://www.asha.org/research/ebp/frame-your-clinical-question/

Bass, R. (1999). The scholarship of teaching: What's the problem? *Inventio: Creative Thinking About Teaching and Learning, 1*(1), 1-10. https://digitalcommons.georgiasouthern.edu/cgi/viewcontent.cgi?filename=0&article=1421&context=ij-sotl&type=additional

Beck, A. R., Seeman, S., Verticchio, H., & Rice, J. (2015). Yoga as a technique to reduce stress experienced by CSD graduate students. *Contemporary Issues in Communication Science and Disorders, 42*(Spring), 1-15. https://doi.org/10.1044/cicsd_42_s_1

Bond, A. R., Mason, H. F., Lemaster, C. M., Shaw, S. E., Mullin, C. S., Holick, E. A., & Saper, R. B. (2013). Embodied health: The effects of a mind–body course for medical students. *Medical Education Online, 18*(1), 20699. https://doi.org/10.3402/meo.v18i0.20699

Friberg, J. C. (2018, February 12). Problems, opportunities, and wonderments: Possible subsets of "what works?" *The SOTL Advocate*. https://illinoisstateuniversitysotl.wordpress.com/2018/02/12/problems-opportunities-and-wonderments-possible-subsets-of-what-works/

George Mason University Writing Center. (2018, August 8). How to write a research question. *Writing Center*. Retrieved 31 January 2022, from https://writingcenter.gmu.edu/guides/how-to-write-a-research-question

Hutcheson, K. A. (2017). Developing a clinical question into a research question: The "use it or lose it" example. *Perspectives of the ASHA Special Interest Groups, 2*(13), 147-154. https://doi.org/10.1044/persp2.SIG13.147

Hutchings, P. (2000). *Opening lines: Approaches to the scholarship of teaching and learning.* Carnegie Foundation for the Advancement of Teaching.

Klopfer, L. (2022, February). Selecting a topic. *Eastern Michigan Library Research Guides.* https://guides.emich.edu/c.php?g=567673&p=3916495

Lieberman, R., Raisor-Becker, L., Sotto, C., & Redle, E. (2018). Investigation of graduate student stress in speech language pathology. *Teaching and Learning in Communication Sciences & Disorders, 2*(2). https://doi.org/10.30707/tlcsd2.2lieberman

Nelson, P., & Goffman, L. (2006). Primer on research: Developing a research question. *The ASHA Leader, 11*(6), https://doi.org/10.1044/leader.FTR3.11062006.15

Oregon Health & Science University. (2022). *Asking your PICO question.* https://libguides.ohsu.edu/nursing/PICO

Price, P. (2013). Section 2.2 Generating good research questions. Accessed April 3, 2023 from http://open.bccampus.ca/find-open-textbooks/?uuid=ef1500d5-fc15-4a36-8d1c-283bf01de2f2&contributor=&keyword=&subject=) and from https://wikieducator.org/index.php?title=ResearchMethods/Introduction/EvalResQues&oldid=987518

Qureshi, F. (2019, February 25). Don't know where to start? 6 tips on identifying research gaps. *Insights.* https://www.editage.com/insights/dont-know-where-to-start-6-tips-on-identifying-research-gaps

Ranganathan, P., & Aggarwal, R. (2018). Study designs: Part 1-An overview and classification. *Perspectives in Clinical Research, 9*, 184-186.

Seppälä, E. M., Bradley, C., Moeller, J., Harouni, L., Nandamudi, D., & Brackett, M. A. (2020). Promoting mental health and psychological thriving in university students: A randomized controlled trial of three well-being interventions. *Frontiers in Psychiatry, 11.* https://doi.org/10.3389/fpsyt.2020.00590

Shah, A. P., & Galantino, M. L. (2019). Building emotional intelligence for student success: A pilot study. *Perspectives of the ASHA Special Interest Groups, 4*(6), 1445-1461. https://doi.org/10.1044/2019_PERSP-19-00101

SUNY Empire State College. (2022). Evaluate your own research question. https://www.esc.edu/online-writing-center/exercise-room/evaluate-your-own-research-question/#:~:text=Evaluate%20the%20quality%20of%20your,question%20easily%20and%20fully%20researchable%3F

University of Michigan Dearborn. (2022). *Advanced psychology research guide.* https://guides.umd.umich.edu/psychology

Vermeesch, A. L., Stillwell, S. B., & Scott, J. G. (2017). Interventions to reduce perceived stress among graduate students: A systematic review with implications for evidence-based practice. *Worldviews on Evidence-Based Nursing, 14*(6), 507-513. https://doi.org/10.1111/wvn.12250

Zope, S. A., & Zope, R. A. (2013). Sudarshan Kriya Yoga: Breathing for health. *International Journal of Yoga, 6*(1), 4. https://doi.org/10.4103/0973-6131.105935

*Note:* The icons used throughout the chapter were created with images from Flaticon.com.

# Worksheet 8-1:
# Developing Your Research Question

| | Gather Grain | Cook | Ferment | Distill | Age | Bottle |
|---|---|---|---|---|---|---|
| **Research** | Read widely | Find the gap | Identify emerging questions | Assess feasibility of questions | Refine question and design study | Conduct research |
| **Questions** | • What do I know?<br>• What do I know about your topic?<br>• What is the foundational knowledge?<br>• What are current trends or directions in this area?<br>• What work seems to be referenced repeatedly? | • What don't I know?<br>• What is missing from the discussion?<br>• What hasn't been explored yet?<br>• What contexts, groups, or views are unexplored?<br>• Are there flaws or missing elements in current studies? | • Could I replicate a study with a different group of people?<br>• Could I conduct a similar study but in a different context?<br>• Should I explore why a correlation exists?<br>• Can I replicate a previous study with a variable change? | • What type of information is needed to answer this question?<br>• Do I have access to participants?<br>• What will the data that I collect look like?<br>• Can I access the technology that I need to conduct this research?<br>• Is timing to conduct study feasible? | • Is my question specific?<br>• Is my question focused?<br>• Is my question worded concisely?<br>• Is my question answerable with measurable or gatherable data?<br>• Is my question complex in nature? | • Complete institutional review board application.<br>• How and where will you recruit participants?<br>• How will you organize, track, and protect data?<br><br>(See Chapter 9) |
| **Ideas** | | | | | | |

# The Process of Conducting Clinical Education Research

*Jayne Yatczak, PhD, OTRL*

It is helpful when engaging in something new to start from a place of familiarity. The process of doing your work as a clinician and the process of doing research have important similarities and differences. They both involve abstract critical thinking and complex reasoning. In clinical practice, and in research, we identify problems or ask questions (reason for client referral, problem statement/research questions), gather information and make observations, develop plans (treatment plan/methodology), and take action (interventions/data collection and analysis). Your knowledge of the clinical process can help you to understand aspects of the research process.

The research process involves the application of various research methods, it requires rigor and control, and outcomes are shared through presentations and publications. There are also other important steps and considerations that you must be aware of when conducting your clinical education research. Obtaining approval to use participants in your research and obtaining informed consent is a necessary and important first step in the process. You will also need to develop a system to manage and ensure the security of your research data. Conducting clinical education research will require you to understand and negotiate the roles and

responsibilities of a clinician/educator/researcher. Taking on these multiple roles and responsibilities will also require you to manage time demands. Conducting your clinical education research will require you to identify and secure any necessary resources. The information provided in this chapter addresses these steps and will help you navigate the process of doing your research. Topics covered in this chapter apply to conducting research in general with an added emphasis on issues related to working with students in your research.

## INSTITUTIONAL REVIEW BOARD

The institutional review board (IRB) may also be called the research ethics board, independent ethics committee, or ethical review board. After you have developed your research idea and written your proposal, the first and most important thing you must do before you can begin your research and engage with your research participants is obtain approval from your IRB. In general, if a study lacks ethics clearance (IRB approval), it cannot be published or publicly presented.

DeRuiter, M., & Ginsberg, S. M. (Eds.). *Clinician's Guide to Applying, Conducting, and Disseminating Clinical Education Research* (pp. 111-122).
© 2024 Taylor & Francis Group.

Going through the IRB process can feel like a daunting step. Some basic information about the why and how will get you through the IRB process and on with your research. It is important to remember that you cannot obtain IRB approval after the fact. If you want to gather data or use student work or assignments, you must plan ahead and get IRB approval before doing so.

The IRB is a committee of at least five people from various backgrounds that has been formally designated by your organization or institution to review and monitor research involving participants. The committee typically consists of individuals with a scientific background, individuals who have expertise and training in nonscientific areas, and members of the community who may represent people who would participate in research studies. The primary purpose of IRB review is to assure, both in advance and by periodic review, that appropriate steps are taken to protect the safety, rights, and welfare of humans partaking as participants in your research. To accomplish the purpose of protecting participants from harm and abuse, IRBs use a group process to review research protocols and related materials (e.g., informed consent documents, interview guides, recruitment scripts). This group review serves an important role in the protection of the rights and welfare of research participants. Kim (2012) has written a brief and interesting review of the historical scandals and social responses to the abuse of participants in research. Her review supports the ongoing need for participants' protection.

The IRB has the authority to approve and require modifications to a research proposal (needed to obtain approval) or disapprove research. It is important to note that your research is limited to what was approved by the IRB. Any changes you make to the study protocol after it has been approved will have to be reviewed and approved by your IRB. Changes could include the risk to participants has changed, you want to modify the design of your study, or you wish to change the consent agreement. Your IRB will have a process for submitting minor and major modifications to your study.

A general understanding of the three ethical principles that are fundamental to participant protection and guide the board's review of your research will be helpful in completing this important and necessary step. The three ethical principles are respect for persons, beneficence, and justice. These are concepts that are probably familiar to you as a clinician. Some aspects of them can be found in most professions' code of ethics. Just as you need to be ethical in your practice, you need to be ethical in conducting your research.

## Box 9-1:
## Ethical Principles of Research

- **Respect for persons:** Addresses the personal dignity and autonomy of individuals, treating them with courtesy and respect and the importance of proper informed consent. Additionally, researchers must be truthful and conduct no deception.

- **Beneficence:** Incorporates the philosophy of "do no harm" and addresses the obligation to protect participants from harm by assessing the risks and benefits of the research and assuring that the anticipated benefits are greater than the anticipated risks.

- **Justice:** Requires that research participants are fairly selected with regard to the purpose and expected outcome of the research and there is an equal opportunity to participate or to not participate. In addition, the population of research participants should be similar to those who may benefit from the outcome of the research.

These ethical principles form the basis for the regulatory standards for participant protection in the United States. The U.S. federal regulations are found in 45 CFR 46 Protection of Human Subjects (U.S. Department of Health and Human Services, 2018). More information on these ethical principles can be found at the Office for Human Research Protections at the U.S. Department of Health and Human Services (HHS. gov) and in the Belmont Report (1979; such as the obligation to obtain informed consent). You may also be able to find guidance on research ethics from your professional organization.

To make sure that you and your research team members are knowledgeable about protecting participants you will be required to complete participants research compliance training and submit proof of completion with your IRB application. Your institution may have a subscription to online compliance training or you can purchase courses for individuals. The Collaborative Institutional Training Initiative and Protecting Human Research Participants provide online regulatory compliance training.

## *Institutional Review Board Review Types*

In navigating the IRB process, it is helpful to know the different types of reviews under which your research may fall. The types of reviews include exempt, expedited, and full board review. The type of IRB review and the associated review process are determined by the:

- Type of research being conducted (e.g., a survey, an ethnographic observation)
- Sensitivity of the research questions or complexity of the research design
- Involvement of vulnerable populations as research participants (e.g., prisoners, children, people with mental disabilities, pregnant women, people with economical and educational disadvantages; 45 CFR §46)
- Use of identifiable information

Most clinical educator research is likely to fall under the exempt category. In general, a study is exempt from IRB review if it is research in commonly accepted educational settings involving normal educational practice. Things like course evaluations, instructional strategies or techniques, or use of educational tools (computer software, apps) would be exempt. Research using surveys, interviews, or questionnaires are also exempt. Observation of public behavior, collection or study of existing data, documents, records, if the sources are publicly available, or if the information is recorded so that participants cannot be identified is exempt. Due to HIPAA, review of medical records are not considered exempt.

When conducting research with students you must be aware of the Family Educational Rights and Privacy Act (FERPA). FERPA (1974; 20 U.S.C. § 1232g; 34 CFR Part 99) is a federal law that protects the privacy of student education records. The law applies to all schools that receive funds under an applicable program of the U.S. Department of Education. Generally, schools must have written permission from the parent or eligible student in order to release any information from a student's educational record. Educational records are directly related to a student. These records include but are not limited to grades, transcripts, class lists, student course schedules, student financial information (at the postsecondary level), and student discipline files. The information may be recorded in any way, including but not limited to handwritten, print, computer media, videotape, audiotape, film, microfilm, microfiche, and e-mail.

Based on your study design and procedures, your IRB will determine if your study is exempt and if there are any FERPA issues. If your research involves educational records, you must adhere to FERPA in addition to IRB decisions. In your IRB application, be very specific about what data you will be collecting. For more information, visit the U. S. Department of Education FERPA website (https://www2.ed.gov/policy/gen/guid/fpco/ferpa/index.html).

It is important to remember that exempt research must be initially reviewed by your IRB. After this initial review, the exempt determination eliminates the need for continuing IRB review and approval. However, you still have an obligation to understand and follow generally accepted principles of responsible and ethical conduct of research. Qualified IRB staff will review your application to determine if it is eligible for exempt status.

Given that most clinical educator research is likely to come under the exempt category, the other types of review will be briefly covered. Expedited reviews are for research that poses a minimal risk and meets one or more of the nine expedited review categories. Most of the expedited review categories pertain to clinical studies of drugs, noninvasive procedures, or collection of biological specimens or blood samples. However, clinical educator research may fall into Expedited Category 6 or Expedited Category 7. Expedited Category 6 includes the collection of data from voice, video, digital, or image recordings made for research purposes. An example would be using video recordings to examine communication styles between educators and students. Expedited Category 7 includes research on individual or group characteristics or behavior (including but not limited to research on perception, cognition, motivation, identity, language, communication, cultural beliefs or practices, and social behavior) or research employing survey, interview, oral history, focus group, program evaluation, human factors evaluation, or quality assurance methodologies.

It would be rare that your clinical educator research would require a full board review. Federal regulations require a full board review for applications where the research involves more than minimal risk to participants. A full board review may also be required when the research involves vulnerable populations (previously listed) or sensitive topics, including illegal behaviors, or the complexity of the research design requires the expertise of multiple board members to evaluate.

## Institutional Review Board Applications

What is in the IRB application? Table 9-1 provides an overview of sections and content required in the IRB application. Informed consent will be covered in greater detail later in this chapter.

How long can you expect the review process to take? Table 9-2 provides general timelines for reviews. You should contact your IRB representative to find out timelines for your setting. Timing of a full board review depends on how often the full board meets. It is important to pay attention to submission deadlines and upcoming IRB meeting dates.

As the researcher, you have a significant influence on the length of time between IRB submission and approval of your research study. There are multiple things you can do to make sure your review goes smoothly and quickly: (1) get to know your research compliance officer (IRB representative) so you can ask questions as you develop your research and before you submit your application, (2) educate yourself on research with participants to help you understand and respect the purpose of the participant review process, (3) take the time to write a well thought out research proposal/protocol (your proposal is where you will get the answers to questions in the IRB application related to the

**Table 9-1**

## CONTENTS OF INSTITUTIONAL REVIEW BOARD APPLICATION

| | |
|---|---|
| General study information | Researcher information, proposed research description, IRB application type (exempt, expedited, full) |
| Where study will be conducted | Describe all sites where the research will take place |
| Study design | Research question, describe the research procedures, describe all interactions with participants |
| Participant information | Target population, recruitment procedures |
| Risks and benefits | Describe risks (physical, psychological, and/or social), precautions taken to minimize risks, describe the anticipated benefits to society and/or individual participants |
| Informed consent | Describe the consent process, upload consent documents |
| Confidentiality, security, and privacy | Indicate identifiability of data, describe privacy protections, data management plan, how data will be kept safe, who will have access to the data, any plans for future use of data |
| Dissemination | Describe plans for dissemination |

**Table 9-2**

## TIMELINES FOR REVIEW

| | |
|---|---|
| Exempt review | 1 week or less |
| Expedited review | 2 to 3 weeks |
| Full board review | 4 weeks or more |

rationale for your research, the target population of your study, recruitment procedures, what you will be asking your participants to do, etc.), (4) make sure you have attached all the essential documents and forms, and (5) respond quickly to IRB requests for revisions, additional information, or documents.

## Informed Consent, Right to Privacy, Protection From Harm

Before involving any people in your research, you must obtain their legally effective informed consent. You must ensure that both aspects of informed consent are met: Participants are "informed" and they "consent." In order for participants to be able to give consent, they must be adequately informed regarding the nature of the research, its purpose, the risks, the benefits, and their privacy. This is the first part of informed consent: the informing process. You will need to allow ample time for the informing process. You should make every effort to be as clear and comprehensive as possible in explaining the research. Allow your potential participants multiple opportunities to ask questions or seek clarification. Provide them with enough time to think about what was presented and give them ample time to consider whether or not to participate. Through the

informed consent process, you have an obligation and an opportunity to enhance the participants' capacity to be self-determining (Sales & Folkman, 2000).

The consent form attests to the fact that the participant is informed about the research for which they are volunteering. It is a written and signed agreement between you, the researcher, and the research participant. It describes the expectations of the participant, as well as the researcher. For example, the research participant might be expected to concentrate on performance tasks being presented or to answer questions as truthfully as possible. You, as the researcher, are expected to carry out the study as it was described in the informed consent process. Table 9-3 has a list of what is included on the consent form.

The language used in the oral and written information about the research, including the written informed consent form, should be nontechnical, jargon-free, and easily understood by the participant. Keep it straightforward and keep it simple. Provide the potential participants with sufficient detail that will help them make an informed decision about whether or not to participate. Kadam (2017) reviewed ways to make the consent process more meaningful, including helpful tips on how to improve the readability of informed consent documents, which includes some of the following: using adequate white space, using lists instead of paragraphs, keeping sentence length below 12 words, and writing the consent form the way you talk.

Not only is informed consent a necessary step in the research process it is also a potential avenue for increasing participation in your research. No matter how great the contribution, your research will make to improving student learning you must get students to volunteer to participate. Indeed, the success of your research hinges on students volunteering for your study. Thomas and colleagues (2019) discussed how to improve participation of students

**Table 9-3**

## WHAT AN INFORMED CONSENT DOCUMENT MUST COVER

1. **Purpose of the study:** This section includes a statement that the study involves research, and in common everyday language, describes why the researcher is doing the study.

2. **Procedures:** This section provides the participant with information about what they will be asked to do and how much time the study will take.

3. **Potential risks and discomforts:** This section describes any potential risks and what the participant can do should any risks or discomfort be experienced during the study.

4. **Anticipated benefits to research participant:** This section describes any benefit that the participant may personally experience as a result of participating in the research study.

5. **Anticipated benefits to society:** Many people choose to participate in research not for personal benefit but to help others. This section describes how the research will benefit others.

6. **Compensation for participation:** This section describes any type of compensation that may be offered to the participant for being in the study.

7. **Identification of investigator:** The name, credentials, and contact information of the principal investigator should be included with instructions to contact them with any pertinent questions about the research, questions regarding the participant's rights, and if there is a research-related injury.

8. **Participation and withdrawal:** This section includes a statement that participation is voluntary and that the participant may refuse to participate in the study or withdraw at any time from the study without penalty.

9. **Consequences of withdrawal:** This section describes what will happen if the participant decides not to continue in the study. It typically includes a statement such as the following, "The participant may discontinue participation at any time without penalty or loss of benefits to which the participant is otherwise entitled."

10. **Privacy and confidentiality:** This section includes a statement regarding the amount of privacy and confidentiality the participant can expect if they choose to participate in the study.

in health professional education research. They advocated for a multifaceted approach that can be used in your clinical educator research. They highlighted the importance of adequate information to allow for students to make an informed choice regarding participation.

Your students may be well educated on clinical research but less familiar with education research. There needs to be clear communication of the research rationale and the potential impact on the clinical experience. Students may be unable to see the relevance or benefit to themselves and other students. This unfamiliarity with education research may require further explanation from you. Partnerships and student co-design of your research is another way to increase meaningful participation and increase students' knowledge and understanding of clinical educator research.

In your efforts to get students to volunteer, it is important to remember that consent must be given voluntarily. Potential participants have the right to consent or to refuse to participate in your research without penalty. It must also be made clear that they may withdraw from the research at any time and for any reason without penalty. You should view informed consent as a continuous dynamic process and not an isolated event that only occurs at the beginning of your study. As you carry out your research, pay attention to any signs that the participant may not want to continue

in the research and make clear that termination of their participation is possible. It is your responsibility to ensure that participation is voluntary and to minimize the possibility of coercion or undue influence in obtaining the initial consent or for ongoing participation.

Coercion occurs if individuals cannot refuse to participate, if refusal results in a substantial loss to the individual, or if individuals believe that participation is not voluntary (Scott-Jones, 2000, p. 29). Coerced consent, either expressed or implied, may occur under a number of circumstances. Doing research with students is one of those circumstances. College students are not designated as a vulnerable population in research. Unlike children and people with mental disabilities, they are able to do a risk/benefit analysis of participation, and unlike prisoners, they are not captive. However, given the importance of engaging in the clinical experience to completing their degree and the potential issues with obtaining another placement, they may feel captive. It is important to keep the issue of coercion in mind as it has the potential to undermine a students' trust in the research process and their trust in you.

A real or perceived potential effect on grades, job recommendations, or career success may influence a students' decision to participate. Students can feel that not participating would reflect poorly on them or that being a good student requires them to participate. Some students may participate to gain your approval. In a review of issues related to students' participation in research, Moorthy (2020) reported that younger students and students of color felt more pressure to participate than their peers. This issue can place a greater burden on disadvantaged students.

It is important to be aware of the power difference between clinical educators and students. Given the power differential between a clinical educator and a student, there exists the very real question, "Is voluntary consent really possible?" Some have argued that using one's own students as research participants is unethical given the power difference (Ferguson et al., 2004). Your process for ensuring consent is voluntary will need to be explained in your IRB application. One common way to address this issue is to have a colleague, research assistant, or a third party not involved in the research obtain consent and hold it until the student has finished the clinical experience.

Offering incentives or inducements is a common practice in research. If you decide to offer inducements for participation, you should be careful to consider the issue of coercion, exploitation, or undue influence. It could be easy to exploit the personal circumstances of students with inducements. Incentives/inducements are anything offered to a potential participant to encourage participation in the research. Inducements often take the form of money or gift cards. An inducement for students could also take other forms such as a schedule change, extra credit, or different assignments.

If you decide to give an inducement for participation and are not sure if it is excessive or could be coercive, seek assistance from colleagues, experienced researchers, or your IRB representative. Remember, there are no hard and fast rules for providing inducements. To avoid any undue influence, consider offering compensation that serves as a "thank you" for participation and a token of appreciation. Any inducements offered for participation should be reviewed as part of your IRB application.

Respect for privacy and confidentiality is another important aspect of conducting ethical research with human participants. The informed consent should contain a statement about the level of privacy participants can expect. Confidentiality refers to the agreement you, as the researcher, has with participants about what may be done with their identifiable private information. This agreement includes how the participants' information is handled, managed, and disseminated. Anonymity means no one can connect the research participant to their data. In clinical education research, it can be difficult to maintain confidentiality and anonymity of data.

In particular, the process of anonymization may be used to protect participants' confidentiality in qualitative research. Frequently, information is recorded in a way that does not link participant responses with identifying information (usually by use of a code known only to the researcher). It may also include giving participants a pseudonym. If you decide to use data that includes a distinctive story that might make a student identifiable, you can change key characteristics of the participant in various ways to disguise the participant's identity. This practice should be done only if it does not affect the integrity of the data (Wiles et al., 2008). Another way to protect participants is to report aggregate findings, not individual-level data.

The privacy and confidentiality of students may not be the only ethical issue when conducting clinical educator research. In addition, depending on your research questions and methodology, you may need to consider the privacy and confidentiality of students' peers, your colleagues, faculty members, clinical coordinators, the educational program, and the educational institution. For example, students could reveal specific information or attitudes about a faculty member who taught the course on how to perform certain clinical tasks. You would want to make sure that the confidentiality of the faculty member is also protected.

Despite being categorized as low-risk, there is the potential for clinical educator research to have unforeseen consequences for students who participate and is something you need to consider. Although physical harm is unlikely to occur, emotional or social harm may occur. For example, students could be embarrassed by their performance, especially if they know that it will be compared to the performances of other students.

## Data Collection, Management, Analysis, and Security

Although methods and aims of research may differ between disciplines, the overall process of data collection is largely the same and is determined by your research question. Data collection is the systematic process of gathering information from various sources. Sources could include observations, interviews, surveys, or specific measurements. The data you collect may be either quantitative or qualitative, depending on the research design (see Chapters 6, 7, and 8). You will collect data based on your proposal and IRB approval. Remember, you can only collect what was approved by your IRB.

Managing research data is an integral part of the research process. Data management requires developing a plan before you collect data and will need to be described in your IRB application. Next to your participants, your data are the most important thing in your research. Through good data management practices, you protect both your data and your participants. The data from your study are crucial as they are the evidence for your results. Data management will reduce the risk of data loss, increase your research efficiency, and protect your participants' information. Data should also be protected for possible future use in verifying the results of your study and for future reanalyzing.

Many of the activities for managing your research data you are already familiar with, such as creating files, naming them so you can find them quickly, backing up data, deleting data that is no longer needed, and controlling who has access to your data. It is important that you keep records secure through the use of password-protected files, encryption when sending information over the internet, and even old-fashioned locked doors and drawers. Properly stored research data ensures that you can maintain the integrity of the data you have collected. Although it seems obvious, do not forget to take the important step of backing up your data, which includes the periodic scanning of any hard copies of data. For a succinct synthesis on research related to qualitative data management, which applies to quantitative data management as well, see Lin's (2009) article.

There are many computer tools available to manage both quantitative and qualitative data. Many of these programs will also assist with data analysis. Using computer-assisted data analysis software will require you to do some investigating into the software best suited to your research needs and your resources. There are several things to keep in mind when choosing a program. Some programs can be quite expensive. However, there are some free programs. Some will assist with analysis of both quantitative and qualitative data, and others are only for use with quantitative or qualitative data. You will also need to consider the ease of use, time it will take for you to learn to use the system, and access to training.

The following are some of the most common programs. Statistical Package for Social Science (IBM) is the most popular quantitative analysis program. Other programs include Statistical Analysis System, STATA, R, and Python. There are many programs for qualitative data analysis software, including ATLASti, MAXQDA, NVivo, QDAMiner, Quirkos, Dedoose, Taguette, and MonkeyLearn.

# Negotiating Roles and Responsibilities

Along with being an educator and a clinician, conducting clinical education research will require you to take on the roles and responsibilities of a researcher. The priorities of each of these roles are different. They often overlap and intersect. However, each role has certain expectations and demands that must be met. You will need to ensure that you meet the demands of your work role, that you focus on student learning while simultaneously maintaining the integrity of your research. The challenge will be for you to meet these demands as you work toward becoming a clinical education researcher.

As an educator, student learning is your number one priority. You are committed to best practices in providing clinical education to your students. Indeed, your commitment to student learning is likely driving your interest in doing clinical educator research. As a clinician, your number one priority is meeting the needs of your clients. Safe and effective treatment is your goal. Quality clinical education can help meet your goal of providing the best care to clients and ensure that students are well prepared to offer the best treatment to their future clients. Finally, as a clinician/researcher, you will want to make sure that gathering data occurs with minimum disruption to client needs. If your research requires observation of student performance, you will need to ask yourself, "How will this interrupt the work of students/will it distress clients?" As a researcher, your priority is in maintaining the rigor and integrity of your research. Your research will serve the important purpose of enhancing student learning, which links back to preparing students for future practice.

You will need to navigate, negotiate, and blend being a clinician-educator, researcher-educator, and researcher-clinician. Arber (2018) discussed how finding this balance between roles was one of the most tiring aspects of being a practitioner-researcher. It may be even more challenging for you given the added role of being an educator. Arber (2018) goes on to discuss how roles and identity can be defined and redefined by oneself and by others. This fluidity of identities can cause discomforting feelings when expectations about identity are not shared at any given moment.

In your role as a clinician, you may experience high clinical service demands. In addition, you have taken on the responsibility of supervising and mentoring students. More than likely, you view your educator role as part of your professional responsibility and a way to give back to the profession. Taking on the role of researcher will add to your already very full professional plate. It is critical to your success to remember that establishing yourself as a clinical education researcher is a process.

Harvey and colleagues (2016) identified four phases in the pathway of becoming a clinician researcher: (1) a research debut, (2) building momentum, (3) developing a track record, and (4) becoming an established clinician researcher. At the end point, research will no longer feel like something separate from or in addition to your work role. Hopefully, it becomes part of the way you and your department do business.

As you first start to develop your research skills, the process will be slow. You need to mentally prepare yourself for this fact. It is easy to feel discouraged when you are used to doing things well and doing them fast. Please remember it took time, commitment, and practice to reach your current level of ability, and with time, commitment, and practice, you will become an established clinical education researcher. If you are reading this book, you probably have the interest and drive to engage in clinical education research. You may also have some of the personal qualities that are leading you to make your research debut. These qualities include natural curiosity, viewing research as integral to being a professional, a desire to improve your educational practice, and a desire to increase your job satisfaction.

## Table 9-4

### ROLES AND RESPONSIBILITIES

| Researcher/ principal investigator | Responsible for all aspects of the study |
|---|---|
| Author of study | Responsible for writing the proposal and connecting the current study to existing studies |
| Methodologist | Responsible for choosing the appropriate methodology to answer the research question |
| Data analyst | Responsible for choosing the appropriate methods for analyzing the data |
| Ethicist | Responsible for the ethical conduct of the research |
| Publicist | Responsible for dissemination of the research |

Remember, your research success will occur progressively, and as you gain experience and develop a track record, you will be in a position to mentor novice researchers. Developing a project that is appropriate to your research skills, gaining organizational support, and developing research relationships will help you develop in your role as researcher. Additional strategies for time management and resources will be discussed later in this chapter.

In order to negotiate the various roles and responsibilities and meet expectations, it is important for you to communicate clearly to students, coworkers, clients, supervisors, and other key stakeholders. It may be harder to clearly communicate about research expectations as you begin your research journey as you may not be entirely clear about research expectations.

Lack of clarity around expectations could lead to potential issues with students, clients, coworkers, and your employer. It will be important for you to make sure that everyone involved in your study knows what is happening, when, and why. The blending of roles can be facilitated by developing scholarship that utilizes your clinical expertise and the creative and effective teaching and learning that already occurs with your students in the clinical setting.

As a clinical educator, you are familiar with balancing the responsibilities of those two roles. Therefore, the rest of this section will focus on the roles and responsibilities of the researcher, the role with which you may be least familiar and comfortable. Faulconer (2021) identified multiple roles within that of the researcher. Within each role comes a set of responsibilities. If you are working on a team, team members may take on some of these roles and responsibilities.

However, you may find yourself filling all of the roles and responsibilities listed in Table 9-4. Each role and its associated responsibilities will be discussed in greater detail.

As the researcher/principal investigator, you are ultimately responsible for the welfare and safety of research participants. The principal investigator also retains responsibility to explain the rationale and the content of the study. Even if other members of your research team are completing the informed consent with participants, you retain responsibility for ensuring that the study is explained in a clear, jargon-free manner and that potential participants are given sufficient time to understand the research and are able to give fully informed consent. As the researcher, you are responsible for supervising any individual to whom you delegate research-related duties and functions (e.g., recruitment of participants, data collection).

As the researcher, you should be qualified by education, training, and experience to assume responsibility for the proper conduct of the research. This workbook can help you prepare to take on the responsibilities of a researcher. The contents of this chapter can help you navigate some of the legal and ethical issues in conducting your research.

As the author of the research study, you will need to ensure that your inquiry is focused on student learning. One way to do this is to include students in the design of your research and have them help develop the research questions. High-quality clinical education research should build upon past published work. You will need to ground your research in past research and enhance the body of evidence through an analysis of previously published work.

As a researcher, you will need to ground your study in the scholarly and local context. Rowlands and Myatt (2013) identified several context questions that should be investigated before you begin your study. These include discussions of why you should do this study and why it is important for various stakeholders (e.g., students, your clinical setting, the educational institution, clients). Finally, you should examine factors that may affect implementation of your study.

Also under the role of researcher are those of methodologist and data analyst. These roles require you to choose sound methodology in the design of your study and choose appropriate ways to analyze the data. You should be thoroughly familiar with the appropriate use of the methods and measures described in your research protocol. Designing a quantitative study was covered in Chapter 6 and designing a qualitative study was covered in Chapter 7.

Being an ethicist involves you conducting your research in partnership with students. It also requires you to educate yourself and follow guidelines for using participants in your research, which was covered in the first section of this chapter.

Your final role is that of publicist. This involves the appropriate dissemination of your research for peer review, critique, and sharing. You may not think this is necessary, but it is an essential step in your research. There are several important reasons to disseminate your research: (1) dissemination increases the credibility of your research, (2) it increases your credibility as a clinical educator, (3) and most importantly, it puts the knowledge gained from your research in the permanent, searchable record. Data that is carefully analyzed and produces new knowledge needs to get to the people that it can help (other clinical educators). Dissemination is also a way to honor the agreement between you and your research participants. Many research participants agree to participate because they believe that by doing so, they will be helping others. Presenting and publishing your work will be covered in detail in Chapters 11 and 12.

## Conflicts of Interest

It is important to know and report any potential conflicts of interest (COIs) that may exist in your research. A COI is not an intrinsically bad thing. The conflict lies in the situation, not in any behavior that you may or may not engage in (Korenman, 2006). Researchers are required to disclose any COIs. Those who need to know about the COI are those who learn about the results of the study and have to interpret it. It is important to report any COI so that it can be evaluated by your audience.

Although money is the most common COI, a COI may also occur when the researcher occupies multiple roles. The one that you need to be particularly aware of is the conflict between being the principal investigator of the research and the clinical educator of the student/participant. You will need to declare your dual role as both a clinical educator and researcher in the information consent letter to the students, even if the activity or exercise to be examined is integrated into regular clinical activities, is of value to study, and involves all students. In clinical education research, the well-being of students and the voluntariness of participation may be compromised by a COI. In addition, the presence of a COI could diminish the credibility of your study. COIs must be managed effectively to maintain the integrity of research, public trust, and the trust of your participants.

## TIME MANAGEMENT AND RESOURCES

In addition to juggling your multiple roles as an educator-clinician-researcher and their unique demands, you will also need to manage your time and identify necessary resources. McKinney (2007) provided two very good reasons for making the time to do research. She advocated that any activity that can improve teaching and enhance student learning is something we should seriously consider. She also suggested that doing research can ultimately save time. Doing clinical education research may help you to be more efficient in how you do clinical education by allowing you to identify and focus on what truly enhances student learning. It may allow you to eliminate tasks or assignments that are less effective in supporting student learning.

The following are some tips to help you manage your time and efficiently move through the research process. First and foremost, pace yourself. Be realistic. It can take a year or more from the time you develop your research question to the dissemination of your research. Another good way to manage your time and support yourself in the process is to integrate your clinical educator research into what you already do as a clinician/educator. In other words, incorporate research into your current practice. Hopefully, you have identified a research question and designed a study that can be incorporated into what you are already doing with your students. Developing a research question was covered in Chapter 8.

Another important strategy is to use teamwork. Collaborating with colleagues, both at the educational institution and in your practice setting, is critical to your work in clinical education research. Collaborating with colleagues, developing partnerships, and sharing expertise can help you move through the research process from start to finish. Remember, many hands make light work. Think broadly about with whom you can collaborate and partner. The best collaborators may be outside your discipline. Indeed, clinical educators from different professions may have the same questions about how to educate students.

Use your newfound knowledge of the roles and responsibilities of a researcher to identify the areas in which you will need help or support. Within each of the roles as researcher and at each step of the research process, there may be people who can help you with some of the work. Partners and collaborators can be an important source of knowledge and expertise. It is especially important to seek out collaborators who have expertise in a particular area in which you do not. For example, you probably do not have the time or desire to become a statistician. You need to partner with or seek out someone who has the statistical knowledge you need for your research.

Do not think of students as only potential research participants. They can also be a great resource. Students can help in the following areas: developing the research question, completing the literature review, collecting data, and analyzing the data. Students as research partners was covered in Chapter 5.

**Table 9-5**

## PHASES OF RESEARCH

| Preliminary phase | Develop research question, literature review |
|---|---|
| Planning phase | Design measures and methodologies, obtain IRB approval |
| Performance phase | Data collection and analysis |
| Final phase | Dissemination |

Mapping out your project can also help you manage your time. It is important to develop a timeline for when each step of the process will be completed. Setting goals and timelines can keep you moving through the process. Understanding what is involved in each phase of the research process can help you estimate the time and resources needed, including reaching out to those who have expertise in different areas. The research process includes the preliminary phase, the planning phase, the performance phase, and the final phase. Table 9-5 provides an overview of the phases. Review Chapters 8 and 10 for a detailed discussion of the full process. A thorough understanding of each phase and what occurs in each phase will not only help you to plan your time and resources but also help you negotiate your multiple roles and responsibilities.

Congratulations! You now know what it takes to make it through the research process and are ready to make your research debut!

# REFERENCES

Arber, A. (2018). Managing the dual identity: Practitioner and researcher. In H. Allan & A. Arber (Eds.), *Emotions and reflexivity in health & social care field research*. Palgrave Macmillan. https://doi.org/10.1007/978-3-319-65503-1_4

Belmont Report. (1979). *The Belmont Report: Ethical principles and guidelines for the protection of human subjects of research*. https://www.hhs.gov/ohrp/regulations-and-policy/belmont-report/index.html

Family Educational Rights and Privacy Act of 1974, 20 U.S.C. § 1232g. (1974). https://www2.ed.gov/policy/gen/guid/fpco/ferpa/index.html

Faulconer, E. (2021). Getting started in SOTL research: Working as a team. *Journal of College Science Teaching, 50*(6), 1-5.

Ferguson, L., Yonge, O., & Myrick, F. (2004). Students' involvement in faculty research: Ethical and methodological issues. *International Journal of Qualitative Methods, 3*(4), 56-68.

Harvey, D., Plummer, D., Nielsen, I., Adams, R., & Pain, T. (2016). Becoming a clinician researcher in allied health. *Australian Health Review, 40*(5), 562-569. https://doi.org/10.1071/AH15174

Kadam, R. (2017). Informed consent process: A step further towards making it meaningful! *Perspectives in Clinical Research, 8*(3), 107-112.

Kim, W. (2012). Review article: Institutional review board (IRB) and ethical issues in clinical research. *Korean Journal of Anesthesiology, 62*(1), 3-12. http://dx.doi.org/10.4097/kjae.2012.62.1.3

Korenman, S. (2006). *Teaching the responsible conduct of research in humans*. Department of Health and Human Services, Office of Research Integrity, Responsible Conduct of Research Resources Development Program. https://ori.hhs.gov/education/products/ucla/default.htm

Lin, L. (2009). Data management and security in qualitative research. *Dimensions of Critical Care Nursing, 28*(3), 132-137.

McKinney, K. (2007). *Enhancing learning through the scholarship of teaching and learning: The challenges and joys of juggling*. Anker Publishing Company, Inc.

Moorthy, G. (2020). Recruiting psychology students to participate in faculty/department research: Ethical considerations and best practices. *Voices in Bioethics, 6*, 1-4.

Rowlands, S., & Myatt, P. (2013). Getting started in the scholarship of teaching and learning. *Biochemistry and Molecular Biology Education*, 1-14.

Sales, B., & Folkman, S. (2000). *Ethics in research with human participants*. American Psychological Association.

Scott-Jones, D. (2000). Recruitment of research participants. In B. D. Sales & S. Folkman (Eds.), *Ethics in research with human participants* (pp. 27-34). American Psychological Association.

Thomas, J., Kuman, K., & Chur-Hansen, A. (2019). Improving the participation of students in health professional education research. *Focus on Health Professional Education: A Multi-Professional Journal, 20*(3), 84-96.

U.S. Department of Health and Human Services. (2018). 45 CFR §46. https://www.hhs.gov/ohrp/regulations-and-policy/regulations/45-cfr-46/index.html

Wiles, R., Crow, G., Heath, S., & Charles, V. (2008). The management of confidentiality and anonymity in social research. *International Journal of Social Research Methodology, 11*(5), 417-428. https://doi.org/10.1080/13645570701622231

# Worksheet 9-1:
# Conducting Your Clinical Education Research

**IRB**

| | |
|---|---|
| Contact information | |
| Timing for reviews | |
| Submission process | |
| Participants training requirement | |

**Informed Consent Considerations**

| | |
|---|---|
| Vulnerable populations or ethical challenges | |
| HIPAA/FERPA information | |
| Identifiable data | |
| Risks to participants | |
| Benefits to participants | |
| Process for reviewing and completing consent | |

Plan to protect data and participant identity:

| |
|---|
| |

*(continued)*

# Worksheet 9-1:
# Conducting Your Clinical Education Research
# (continued)

Potential COIs:

|  |
|--|
|  |

**Timeline for Research**

| Phase | Activity | Time Frame |
|-------|----------|------------|
| Preliminary | Develop research question, literature review |  |
| Planning | Design measures and methodologies, obtain IRB approval |  |
| Performance | Data collection and analysis |  |
| Final | Dissemination |  |

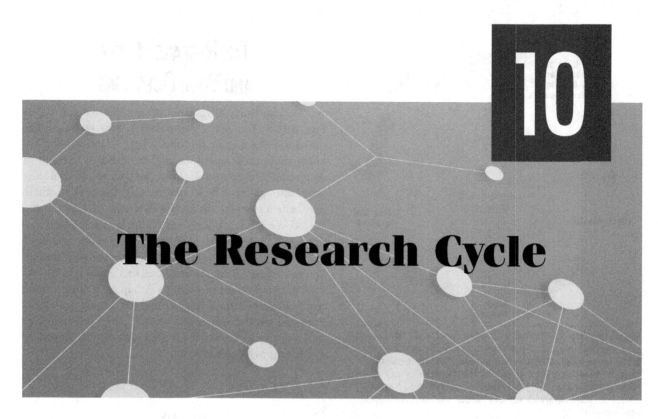

# The Research Cycle

*Mark DeRuiter, MBA, PhD, CCC-A/SLP, F-ASHA*

You may have heard people say that you need a research doctorate (PhD or EdD) to conduct research. This is a myth. Holding a research doctorate isn't a minimum requirement for conducting research. While there are many benefits of doctoral education, you can still do research without it. One of the keys to being successful to conducting research is regularly accessing feedback and gaining the perspectives of other thinkers, as you do during guided research, such as a thesis or dissertation. Similarly, there are fellowship programs offered by organizations large and small that can be valuable because they build in a structure that gives you regular interactions and feedback with professionals who have more experience than the participants themselves. While we can't provide you with a fellowship or a doctoral education in this workbook, we have tried to give you some of the background knowledge and structure that parallels formal mentorship and educational programs—albeit in compressed and miniature form. This chapter will also help you develop a pattern of getting feedback throughout your process.

In Chapter 5, you read about developing a board of mentors. The concepts presented here will be more successful if you have given thought to that board of mentors and are able to gather them as you start your journey into research. We suggest that research is a cycle.

Thinking about research as cyclical can be something that is useful to you as you read the last few chapters of this workbook. As you read through this chapter, you'll find that some elements of the research cycle will encourage you to reflect back on previous things you've read. At other points, the conversation will take you to what is yet to come in the workbook. We encourage you to connect what you have learned and what you recognize you need to continue learning about with how you can learn the information along the steps of the cycle. This chapter will serve as a great way for you to pull all elements together—consider it your bridge to the final chapters.

DeRuiter, M., & Ginsberg, S. M. (Eds.). *Clinician's Guide to Applying, Conducting, and Disseminating Clinical Education Research* (pp. 123-131).

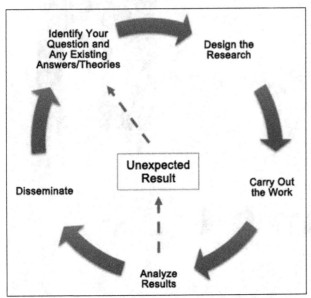

**Figure 10-1.** The research cycle. (Adapted from Loma Linda University School of Dentistry. [n.d.]. *Student research cycle*. Retrieved August 4, 2022, from https://dentistry.llu.edu/research/student-research/student-research-cycle and University of Warwick Policy and International Studies. [n.d.]. *The research cycle*. Retrieved August 4, 2022, from https://warwick.ac.uk/fac/soc/pais/research/csd/teaching/iatl/process/)

## BEGINNING WITH YOUR QUESTIONS

Research begins with asking questions (Vale, 2013). You might have a myriad of questions that you want to ask about clinical education or other topics for that matter! Sometimes, the answers to our questions are easily answered. When things are simple, you can quickly pick up your smartphone, conduct an internet search, and find just what you need to know. However, there are many other times where the answers are a lot less clear. And that is what this workbook is all about. For instance, you are looking for answers to your questions about an issue you are having with clinical education with a graduate physical therapy student and you are working in a free-standing rehabilitation program. As you start to peruse the literature, you find some information in the literature about a similar issue with undergraduate nursing students in a hospital. You might find the knowledge in that article helpful, but it might leave you with some unanswered questions due to the differences in context and educational experience level. You feel that the scenarios are different enough that you need to look further for answers that are more germane to your context. This is where your questions start to grow and you begin to think about how to get reasonable answers that could assist you and others.

## THE RESEARCH CYCLE AND YOUR QUESTIONS

We can think of research on a cycle like you see in Figure 10-1. This figure demonstrates how we might ask questions (starting in the upper left), examine what we know about those questions, and then design research to determine further answers. Once we have found some answers through research, we disseminate that work so others may benefit from our discovery. Then, the cycle continues.

As you know, it's likely not as simple as something like this figure makes it appear. To answer questions, you need to be very thoughtful and do a high degree of planning. You've discovered this throughout this workbook as you consider your board of mentors (Chapter 5), institutional review boards (IRB; Chapter 9), and developing your questions and research design (Chapter 8). There are many elements to consider, and usually your ideas can be shaped by conversations along the way.

### BOX 10-1: YOUR BOARD OF MENTORS

Although your board of mentors was covered in Chapter 5, we want you to consider that group of people again in the context of this chapter. It's impossible to know everything! Make sure your board of mentors contains a wide range of people who have varied expertise. Nothing is more invigorating than having a mentor say, "Have you considered …" and they pull forward some entirely new and helpful information for you!

## PUTTING THE RESEARCH CYCLE TO WORK

Now, take a look at Figure 10-2, which is an adaptation of Figure 10-1. You'll use this figure as you step through the next sections of this chapter, and it will give you an opportunity to take some notes. You'll see that some of this information is consistent with what you have read in other chapters. This is your opportunity to pull it all together—while considering that the research cycle never ends! Let's get going and step through each area of the cycle.

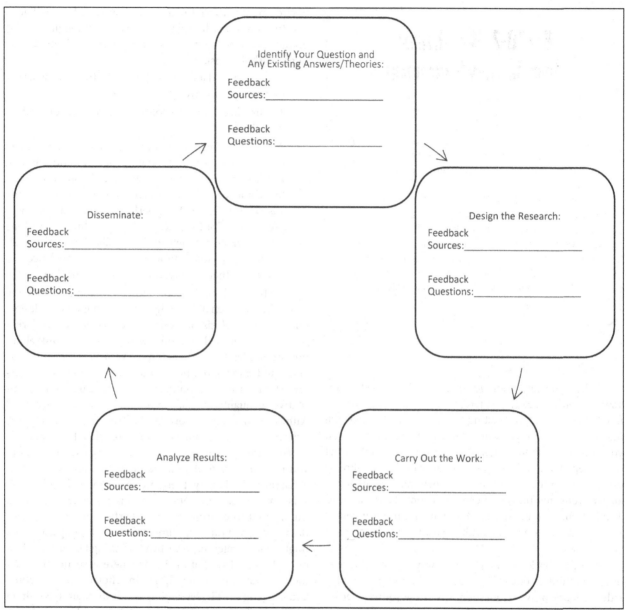

**Figure 10-2.** The research cycle adapted for clinical educator reflection. (Adapted from Loma Linda University School of Dentistry. [n.d.]. *Student research cycle*. Retrieved August 4, 2022, from https://dentistry.llu.edu/research/student-research/student-research-cycle and University of Warwick Policy and International Studies. [n.d.]. *The research cycle*. Retrieved August 4, 2022, from https://warwick.ac.uk/fac/soc/pais/research/csd/teaching/iatl/process/)

## *Identify Your Question and Any Existing Answers/Theories*

So where do you begin? You might be tempted to look at your own discipline first to determine what we already know. We will encourage you to do so! However, don't rule out what we might know from other fields as well. For instance, if you are interested in simulation in occupational therapy, you might find reasonable answers scouring literature in occupational therapy, physical therapy, nursing, and medical education literature (to name a few). Make sure to check journals, books, professional associations, and more. Sometimes you will stumble upon just the right information through a scan of references—something discussed in Chapter 8.

After you have taken time to review the literature, you'll see that your remaining questions start to take shape, but perhaps in a way that requires some edits. We call this *refining your question*.

## Feedback Sources and Questions

When you find your questions aren't completely answered, you are ready to identify and draft your final refined question and the existing information associated with it. Ask yourself who you know (or would like to ask, even if you don't know them) about this question. Remember that it is acceptable to ask people you haven't met but who are doing work in the area of interest. They might be happy to answer your questions and engage in some brief dialogue. Think about what questions are still in your mind and what you would like some help with regarding the direction of your question.

Now, go back to Figure 10-2. As you consider your question, think about what sources you might use to provide feedback on your question. Are these sources people on your board of mentors? Others? (You could even include other resources here, such as books, journals, or websites). And what questions do you have? Take a little time to fill out the blanks in Figure 10-2 so that you don't lose track of your thoughts.

## *Design the Research*

Once you have refined your questions, you might develop some hypotheses. For instance, maybe you want to know more about how students incorporate types of feedback in a given clinical environment. You might hypothesize that orally reported feedback has a greater influence on growing clinicians than written feedback with no explanation. This could be something you test in an appropriate environment with well-planned measures. All this will lead you to how you will design your work. Although we can't predict every element of your design, some elements you might wish to consider are:

- The types of data you will be collecting and whether they are quantitative, qualitative, or both.
- The use/necessity of a control group, dependent upon your design.
- Any environmental manipulations you might need to make for meaningful data collection and analysis. For instance, you might need to add additional time to a clinical day for the student consent process, as discussed in Chapter 9. Or perhaps you are delivering a specific type of feedback to a novice clinician and the time at which you deliver that feedback is a critical element of the study. In a case like this, you'll need to make sure that you are available to get this done.

All this leads you to considering research design on the whole. You've been able to engage with chapters on design, quantitative analysis, and qualitative analysis. Considering what you've learned along the way, you could think about how design leads to the analysis of your data. For instance, you could think about using your data to describe the current status of a situation. Here you might use your quantitative or qualitative data to describe where things stand within the discipline. Correlational research will help you determine if two or more variables are related in some way. Often, using quantitative data here is very useful to you as you run analyses to determine the nature and strength of a relationship. Finally, there are experimental and quasi-experimental design options. In this instance, you might think about comparing groups of participants who are randomly assigned into experimental/control groups, and you might start scratching your head thinking about the ethics of a situation like that. If that is where your mind is racing to—bravo! You will find that in scholarship of teaching and learning (SoTL) research it can be difficult to withhold what you deem might be "good teaching" from a group, simply for the purposes of an experiment.

What you've read in the previous paragraph is helpful, but on a higher level. We'd like to nudge your thinking to something even more granular here as you consider your work. When you think about conducting research in teaching and learning, you might also consider these elements in your design:

- Efficacy of approach (this is often examined using things like labs/simulations where learners engage, and their learning/experience is evaluated by the researcher). Here you could consider things like measuring knowledge and/or skill pre-/post-intervention. You could use your quantitative analysis toolbox, tools from your qualitative box, or mix your methods.

# Box 10-3:
## Mixed-Method Design

Mixed-method research design is exactly what you think it is: research that includes both qualitative and quantitative data being collected and analyzed. This can be daunting for new researchers because it means that you have to understand two different methodologies, but folks on your board of mentors might be able to help you navigate this design.

Typically, in mixed-method research, one data collection approach leads the researcher into the other data collection approach. Which approach leads and which follows can vary. Here are two examples:

1. Quantitative, qualitative: You administer a survey (quantitative) to an entire group of students who completed a semester of clinical practicum in the same hospital unit. After receiving the survey results, you decide you want to learn more about why participants answered the way they did, so you invite them to participate in individual interviews (qualitative) to talk more about their responses on the survey.

2. Qualitative, quantitative: You would like to develop an assessment tool that will measure student learning based on characteristics of your clinical setting. However, you are not sure which parameters might be most important to include in the assessment tool. You arrange a focus group (qualitative) with participants to learn more about what aspects of the clinical setting were salient and relevant to their learning. Based on these data, you create an assessment tool (quantitative) that is targeting the elements that are most likely to be relevant.

---

- Effectiveness data (real-world/real learner-based). In this instance, we think about what might "work best" in a real-world situation. This area might be very appealing to you if you are an active clinical educator. As before, you might use quantitative, qualitative, or mixed designs. However, you need to consider your real-world environment and what may or may not be feasible. This might influence both your design and your question.

- Implementation studies (this research is designed to look at how we get best practice-/evidence-based education adopted into a specific context or type of setting). As you think about this area, you might see some similarity or overlap with the category before. However, what you want to consider here is how you might take what you have learned from both of the study types discussed earlier and actually get them brought into use in a setting. For instance, consider the previous example about delivering feedback to novice clinicians. Imagine you conduct multiple studies across several environments over time and determine that there really is a best way for learners to have feedback delivered to them to learn most effectively. It might be time to take this work into the community and move it forward as a best practice in your community settings. Doing so gives you a wide variety of ways to collect data as you implement the work and further research the implementation of the new feedback method across a variety of appropriate settings.

All these areas of design will require careful thought, and they are based on the principles of implementation science (which is beyond the scope of this chapter). However, if you'd like to learn more, reading Bauer and Kirchner (2020) can be an excellent start.

# Box 10-4: Leaning on Your Board of Mentors for Design and Beyond

You'll need to continually go back to your questions and determine what is feasible given your time, environment, and resources. Don't hesitate to rely on your board of mentors as you move this ahead. Talk with them about what your ideas are for design and how the research would be situated in the realm of efficacy, effectiveness, and implementation research. What questions do you have that they could help you with—ranging from the feasibility of your study being conducted to the relative rigor that it will have as judged by others? You want to be sure that your research is well-designed and without critical flaws.

Take a moment to reflect back on Figure 10-2 and determine where your feedback sources and questions might be—just like you did earlier. Remember, you might need to even move beyond your board of mentors for some feedback, and this is appropriate. Perhaps a member of your board can give you a warm handoff with an appropriate introduction to an expert.

## Carry Out the Work

This is often the exciting part! You will be working with your subjects and collecting data along the way. You'll want to be sure that all the things you have planned are working to make sure there are no areas that you have inadvertently overlooked or forgotten. For instance, if you are conducting an electronic survey, you'll want to confirm that the data are coming in as expected and are something you can export from any software you are using. Note, by "the data are coming in as expected," we don't mean that you are continually confirming whether or not the data are fitting any hypothesis or preconceived notions you may have. Instead, make sure that all the data are collected and secure. Take this example from survey research: Imagine you've developed a 20-question survey. As the data are being collected, you notice that no respondents are replying to questions 13 through 16. Why is that happening? Is this something you might expect? Or is it a glitch in your survey? Talking with your mentor(s) as you are in the midst of this process can provide you with reassurance that you are headed in the right direction, or may provide you with course correction so that any obstacles you might face are not detrimental to the quality of your work.

As you move into the phase where you carry out your work, you will want a place to take some notes and be ready to ask questions as you move along. It might be a little far ahead for you to fill this in on Figure 10-2, but you might also already have some musings about carrying out the work (e.g., Where will I securely hold the data? Who will have access to the data? How will I have enough time in my day to get this work done?). Questions like these are appropriate to consider as you move ahead with this next stage in your thinking. You'll have a chance to reflect on this in the worksheet at the end of the chapter, too.

## Analyze Results

This can sometimes feel like a daunting area. Chapters 6 and 7 were written with a mind toward getting you to think about qualitative and quantitative data collection. However, you'll rely on other sources as well. Our best advice is this: If you have the luxury of working with a statistician for quantitative analysis, make contact with that person as you design your work. It will make the analysis phase that much easier for you because your statistical consultant can guide you not only in the type of data to collect but what you might do with it as a first pass immediately after it is collected. Make sure to take your time with analysis. Errors here can be costly and embarrassing. Your mentors can be invaluable to you here. You may want to have them review your analysis and serve as peers to validate your analyses of the data (within the confines of your IRB proposal). Make sure to check and cross-check each other as you move through the analysis process. You should develop a culture where there is no harm nor foul calling out an error in analysis. Instead, you are all protecting your research interests and credibility!

If qualitative analysis is your game, consider your questions carefully and determine who might serve on your board of mentors who can help you think through the analysis before you even start the work. Some of the best qualitative research can be delayed because you do not have the time or resources to analyze all the data you have collected. Think about the volume of data and future work with a qualitative analysis and how you might develop a team of people to help you carry out the work of the analysis. You might consider how your research could be "chunked" into several different questions that require analysis. This could give you an opportunity to answer one question at a time in your analysis phase, giving you work to disseminate orally or in writing as you move along.

Now, take a moment to head back to Figure 10-2. Think about your future analyses and what questions and feedback might be required. A little planning can take you a long way! Where are you going and who do you need on your team?

## Disseminate

Take yourself back to Chapter 4 of this book. Here we reflected on McKinney's hierarchy, which involved a base of good clinical education, followed by scholarly clinical education, and then the SoTL in clinical education. In this hierarchy, we started with clinicians doing "good work" and moved from there to "doing good work, informed by evidence" (McKinney, 2007). However, you are now at the point of thinking about the SoTL within clinical education if you are holding data in your hands (or computer!) that might inform the process of clinical education. This is an exciting place to be—and it is your responsibility to spread the word! In Chapter 1, we defined the SoTL this way:

> SoTL refers to a body of research that informs best practices in higher education. It can be described as systematic, high-quality research that informs us of the best practices for education. SoTL research examines learner characteristics, teaching approaches, and the context of teaching and learning. By conducting and reading this type of research, we learn about the best ways in which to prepare future clinicians.

Presenting and publishing are areas critical to the research process, and they are what helps define SoTL on the whole. An altruistic way of thinking about it is like this: Once you have collected your data, how can what you have learned help others? It is only going to be through dissemination of the information to your peers. There can be a variety of ways to do this— through posters, oral presentations, blogs, newsletters, books, and peer-reviewed publications. Dependent upon where you work, some of these venues might be more highly valued than others.

But how will you do this? Part of it depends upon beginning with the end in mind. Perhaps you started out thinking about who should know about your work and why it might be important. This is great, and something we encourage. However, sometimes you find other new and exciting elements that might shift or widen your audience for your work. Your mentors might have ideas about how to approach different venues or how to adapt your work to reach a variety of readers or conference attendees. Talk with them about how to get as much variety and value out of your work as you can.

Chapters 11 and 12 are written with dissemination as the end in mind. Make sure to look at them closely as you make your plans for the future.

Finally, remember that you started off with questions you were asking as you began data collection. However, sometimes we have some surprising findings along the way. For instance, maybe you conducted a mixed-method design. Your quantitative analysis seems to bear out your original thoughts and you think, "Excellent! I am proving my hypothesis!" However, when you delve into the qualitative analysis, you learn that there was a third, unexpected variable at play that you hadn't considered. This doesn't need to be the end of the line—simply something that you consider as you disseminate your work. Another way the answers to our questions might drift is that sometimes we see that we might have changed the design of our work, had we known a specific change might happen in the environment, but it's too late to make a change. An example might be that your work was cut short because of changes in staffing in a clinical environment, but the analysis of the data still "fits" the question you were asking. This might lead you to question, "Is the time period I was considering necessary?" All these things are not catastrophic. Instead, they are part of the research arc—you ask questions and you find many more to answer along the way. This can feed a line of research over time! Take yourself back to Figure 10-1 and you'll see something near the center of the circle—a way to think about what happens when things don't turn out as planned! Your analysis can simply feed the question cycle.

## Dissemination Continued: Consider Your Audience

Although you might find hearing about it many times a bit tiring, beginning with the end in mind will be important relative to your audience as well. As you ask your questions and collect your data, you should continually be asking yourself, "Who needs to know about this? What audience will find it important?" Then, you might want to step back and think about your answer to that question. Could there be a broader audience than the one you are considering? For instance, as a physical therapist, you might be asking great questions relative to clinical education. That work might be very important to both academicians and clinicians in physical therapy. However, is that your only audience? Could occupational therapists, speech-language pathologists, or respiratory therapists (to name a few) find your work important as well? It is possible and something to strongly consider as you move forward. It could be useful for you to step outside of your comfort zone and get yourself in front of other audiences/in different venues along the way.

We will have more to say about these venues and audiences in Chapters 11 and 12. For now, just remember it might be tempting to start blogging about your work to share it widely. The caution there is that a journal or other publisher might ask how your work has been disseminated and if it is available elsewhere. You'll want to cautiously consider where people can find your research and how that contributes to your own goals very carefully!

## Other Considerations Within Dissemination

There is certainly a lot to think about when disseminating your work. We'd be remiss if we didn't give you a few other suggestions to consider along the way. Take a look at the box in this chapter for other frequently asked questions. Also, reflect back on Chapter 5 where mentorship was discussed by Lizbeth H. Finestack. Remember, having a strong board of mentors will be of great assistance to you—and it could save you a great deal of time!

Now, take a look back at Figure 10-2. What questions and feedback come to mind as you consider dissemination? We've certainly given you a lot to think about! Take a moment to document them now, while they are fresh in your mind.

# FINAL THOUGHTS

This chapter gives you a broad overview of the research cycle. For some of it, you might say, "I think I've seen this before," and for other areas, you might think, "Well, I need to learn more about that before I move forward." This chapter is an excellent point to get you looking both forward and backward in time. Congratulations on making it this far—and remember that spending some time reflecting back, as well as considering the future, can be very useful!

## Box 10-5:
## Frequently Asked Questions About Research Dissemination

Q: I want to present at a conference, but not all my data are collected yet. Is that acceptable?

A: It could be. You'll want to consider several things: Look closely at the call for papers and determine if there are instructions from the conference organizers regarding research in process. Make sure to follow the directions and do not make conclusions about data you have not analyzed. When presenting the data, make sure it is clear to your audience that your work is not complete!

Q: I wanted my community to know about my research, so I created a blog where I published all my data. I am now writing it up for a journal article and one question from the publisher is: Has this work been published elsewhere? Can I take down the blog and say, "No"?

A: We do not advise that you do this. Instead, have a conversation with the publisher/editor about the work and work with the advice they provide to you.

Q: I've always heard that "negative results" aren't publishable. I did some work, but my hypotheses weren't proven. Does this mean I wasted my time?

A: Not necessarily! Think of the SoTL community as one that is learning and growing along with you. Think about what you *did* learn from your work and how it might be useful to others. It could be worth a conversation with a conference organizer or journal editor to see if there is a place for your work.

Q: I work in a university setting. My mentor there said that SoTL work might not get me tenure or promotion. Is that true?

A: This is a broader institutional and intellectual community discussion. We believe, firmly, that research surrounding teaching and learning *is* research and has value. However, you will want to carefully evaluate the advice you receive in this process to make sure it aligns with your career goals.

Q: I have ways to look at data and disseminate it, but I never got an IRB for the process. What should I do?

A: Before spending a great deal of time with these data, you need to check with your IRB (see Chapter 9). You do not want to spend time with data you cannot ethically disseminate. Remember, many journals will ask you if you have followed the IRB process at the point of submission for a potential publication.

Q: My conference presentations/publications have been rejected. What am I doing wrong?

A: Although we cannot advise every situation with one simple answer, look closely at any feedback you have received. Haven't gotten any feedback? Ask for it! Typically, rejections around publication will have a clear response, but those regarding a presentation might not. It's possible that a conference organizer can provide you with information that is very helpful in guiding your future research or where you might submit in the future.

Q: You say to "begin with the end in mind," but I don't even know that end. Help!

A: Here is where your board of mentors is critical (see Chapter 5). If you find that your mentors aren't able to assist, it might be time to consider expanding your board.

## References

Bauer, M. S., & Kirchner, J. (2020). Implementation science: What is it and why should I care? *Psychiatry Research, 283*, 1-6. https://doi.org/10.1016/j.psychres.2019.04.025.

McKinney, K. (2007). *Enhancing learning through the scholarship of teaching and learning: The challenges and joys of juggling.* Anker.

Vale, R. D. (2013). The value of asking questions. *Molecular Biology of the Cell, 24*(6), 680-682. https://doi.org/10.1091/mbc.E12-09-0660

# Worksheet 10-1:
# The Research Cycle

**Identify Your Question and Any Existing Answers/Theories:**

Feedback
Sources:_____

Feedback
Questions:_____

**Design the Research:**

Feedback
Sources:_____

Feedback
Questions:_____

**Disseminate:**

Feedback
Sources:_____

Feedback
Questions:_____

**Analyze Results:**

Feedback
Sources:_____

Feedback
Questions:_____

**Carry Out the Work:**

Feedback
Sources:_____

Feedback
Questions:_____

Who on your board of mentors might give you useful feedback and insights before you consider presenting?

What kind of feedback would you like to receive before moving forward with your research at each stage?

11

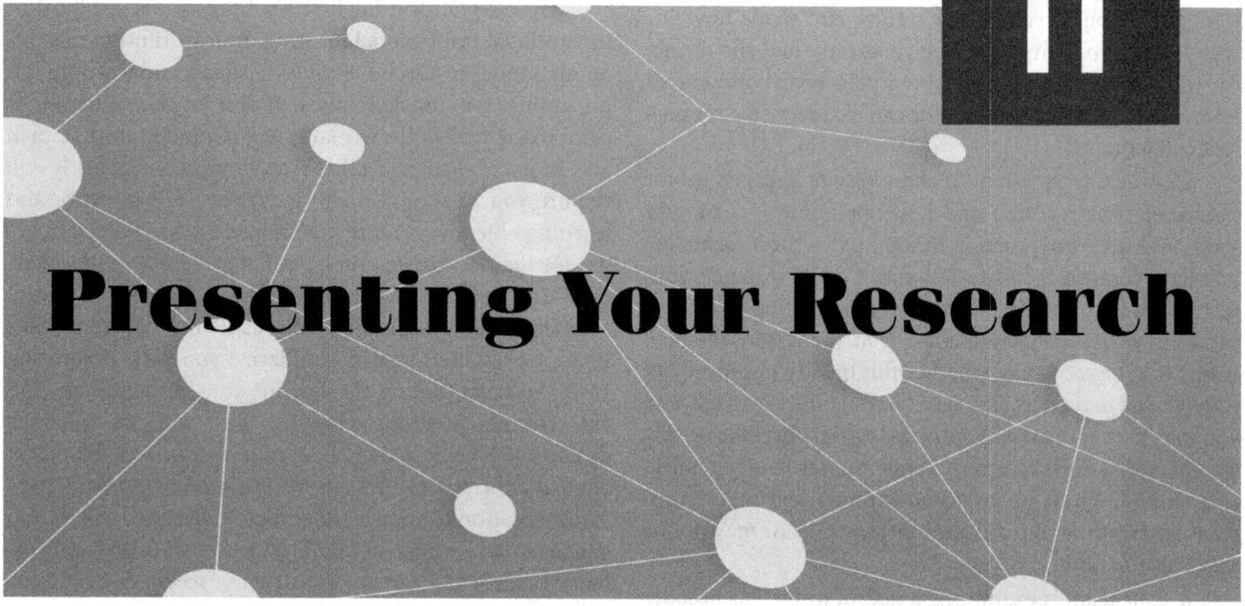

# Presenting Your Research

*Elizabeth A. VandeWaa, PhD*

The scientific method, the mainstay of evidence-based education-clinical education, results in the same outcome, no matter the discipline: *dissemination of results.* In this chapter, we will review how to present results through an oral presentation or a poster. We will include discussion of how your audience shapes your presentation as we examine several different types of opportunities for sharing your professional expertise.

The importance of knowledge dissemination cannot be overstated. If you have discovered something new and relevant in your discipline that may be helpful to clients, clinicians, or students of the discipline, it benefits the wider community of your colleagues and students to share those results. But if you are new to presenting, it may seem like a daunting task. It is well-known that public speaking ranks high on the list of "most terrifying activities" for people. In this chapter, we will discuss methods whereby you may take the fear out of presentation, while charting your path to becoming a polished expert in your field.

## Your Presentation: The Audience and the Contents

As you begin your professional career, you may identify questions that pique your interest and require investigation. You may have colleagues or professional contacts who share your interest and would like to participate in research. If you are new to the process of research, it is advantageous to partner with a more seasoned colleague who has published and presented in your (or a related) discipline. To start, you may engage with other colleagues inside your facility to examine a research question. You may also want to invite professionals from other institutions who may have interest in the issue—these may be individuals with whom you have worked (or attended graduate programs) in the past. Finally, consider adding professional colleagues outside of your discipline if it is determined that your research question has interdisciplinary ramifications. The team with



DeRuiter, M., & Ginsberg, S. M. (Eds.). *Clinician's Guide to Applying, Conducting, and Disseminating Clinical Education Research* (pp. 133-143).
© 2024 Taylor & Francis Group.

which you work will help shape your audience as you collect data and prepare it for dissemination. If you find yourself undertaking research on your own, seek out a trusted mentor with experience to help frame your research question, guide you as you gather results, and shape how you will present your findings. You've already had the chance to read Chapter 5 and think about your board of mentors. Remember, sometimes a mentor can also serve as an excellent collaborator.

How and with whom to share results depends on the nature of your research and how applicable it is to your scope and sphere of practice. In some cases, the information you have gleaned is institution-specific. For instance, your institution may be implementing a new staffing procedure or using novel instrumentation. You (and your research team) may be recording whether this quality improvement is beneficial to novice clinicians learning the approach, and you may have framed a hypothesis to assess benefits vs. disadvantages to their learning. While the results you collect may provide guidance to administrators and other clinicians and staff in your institution, they may or may not be applicable to others.

If your team is examining a question that has broader implications for your profession—either in your geographic location, nationally or globally—the audience that may find these results useful will grow. Additionally, if your team is interdisciplinary, there may be professionals in multiple fields who may find the information relevant, expanding the audience even more.

# Contexts for Dissemination of Results

There are several opportunities for data dissemination in the clinical sciences. Professional meetings may be local, regional, national, or international. Additionally, they may be "live" in a face-to-face format or convene virtually. Your presentation may be synchronous or asynchronous, as part of a panel discussion, group, or as a solo presentation. The format of your presentation may be an oral speech or a poster. The format, length of presentation, and audience type will depend on the setting, but all professional settings will have audience members consisting of participants of varying ranks, stages of career, and disciplines. Targeting your presentation to fit your audience is a key to successful presenting.

As you prepare any presentation, remember it is an opportunity to engage your colleagues and peers in evidence-based education. You will be the expert of the content you will present—this is always a confidence boost for anyone who disseminates results.

## Local-, State-, or Institution-Based Presentations

A good platform for first-time presenters is a local or institutional professional meeting. Your institution may offer an annual research forum or teaching and learning opportunities for clinicians and staff over lunchtime breaks or prior to the start of the workday (e.g., Grand Rounds, Lunch and Learn). Local professional chapter meetings likely will require you to submit a short abstract of your work and learning objectives. These meetings are a good place to begin for the novice presenter, particularly in the early phases of data collection or when the project is in a formative state in the feedback cycle, as discussed in Chapter 10. This type of presentation will familiarize you with organizing your thoughts, timing the flow of your presentation, and entertaining questions regarding your work. It will help develop the central theme of your work—is it based on clinical educator needs? An institutional or learning gap? A presentation to your work or local colleagues will let you gauge audience interest and engagement. Further, this offers an excellent forum for constructive feedback from your colleagues.

As your hypothesis gels and data collection is nearly finished or actively occurring, it may be time to present your findings to a state organization in your discipline. At this stage of your research process, your data will either support your study question—or it may not. Do not consider "negative" data or an unsupported hypothesis to be of no scientific use. Presenting findings of what does not work, or what clinicians previously thought was useful—and now has been discounted by your work—is important. It may not be without controversy and detractors, so make sure you have the evidence—either supported by literature from peer-reviewed sources or from your own research—to support your findings.

The duration of an oral presentation in your institution or at a state or chapter meeting will typically be dictated by the meeting planner. Most often, you may find that you have a short time to get your points across (15 minutes). If you are given a longer time frame, use it as an opportunity to build a case for your work. As you prepare, make sure you have relevant references and background that is appropriate for your audience. Common components of presentations are discussed later in this chapter.

## National or International Presentations

A presentation to a statewide organization may fuel the interest of those in your discipline in such a way that there is impetus for you to present the data nationally. The national meeting may be in your area of clinical expertise or in that of other collaborators on your project. If you are attending a national meeting, there is much to know! First, you will have to submit an abstract and objectives of your presentation. Typically, the collaborator who has the most expertise relative to the conference will be the lead on the abstract. For instance, if you are working with a nurse on a project that highlights issues of teaching patient medications and the abstract is submitted to a nursing conference, the nurse collaborator would likely be the lead and the contact person. Once submitted, a committee for the organization will read your abstract and objectives, deciding on the validity and soundness of the presentation, as well as prospective audience member interest in the topic. Accepted abstracts will often be printed in proceedings of the meeting. If the abstract was peer-reviewed prior to acceptance, this could be included on your professional curriculum vitae. You will be notified of acceptance of your abstract, and the format in which the organization will want the information presented. Presentation formats are typically a poster session or an oral talk. Regardless of the format, the sponsoring organization will need a description of your talk, the technology you intend to use, and other paperwork that will require a timely response. Make sure you adhere closely to the deadlines the organization posts.

Acceptance of your abstract to a national or international conference is an indicator of the quality and rigor of your work. These conferences represent the pinnacle of knowledge dissemination in the sciences. Recognize that they may have costs you have not considered outside of travel, including registration, society membership, and additional fees for presentations you may wish to attend. As you plan your travel, these costs plus time off from work may be prohibitive. Your employer may sponsor some or all the cost of attendance, but this is not an automatic when presenting at meetings.

# TYPES OF PRESENTATIONS

## *Posters*

A poster presentation may be a good first step at a national or international conference. It will allow you to familiarize yourself with how the conference is run, while assessing learner interest in your research topic. Poster sessions often require the presenter to be standing at the poster for an hour or more. Make sure you attend the complete duration of your session, no matter how many (or how few) attendees there are. Presenting a poster provides a "lower stakes" interaction with conference attendees. You will be able to chat one-on-one or with a small group of professionals. Rehearse the salient points of your poster to share with those who stop to consider it—leading the conversation will help engage the attendee. The cordial atmosphere of poster presentations often puts novice presenters at ease, although colleagues may still ask challenging questions.

Engage learners by being an active listener, receiving their input and criticisms with an open mind. Use body language and facial expressions that indicate your openness to comments and constructive feedback. Speak with enthusiasm and passion about your project, without engaging in rancorous discourse.

Remember, a poster is not the same as a paper. You will not include all the details of a paper or your research. The purpose of a poster session is to present a visually engaging representation of your work. It should give the viewer an overview of what you did, how you did it, and what you learned. Think of the poster as a conversation starter. It is common for a conference attendee to approach a poster, read it quickly, and then turn to the presenter to engage in dialogue about the work. If you have too much text in the poster, it will take too long for the attendee to read and process. Many conference attendees will be dissuaded from reading a very lengthy and text-heavy poster, as they usually have a handful of posters and presenters they want to see all in the same time frame. There are some great resources available online that might be useful to you for creating attractive posters (New York University, 2022; Pinch, 2022). Please see the References list for more helpful materials.

## Poster Presentation Guidelines

Many online resources will allow you to construct a poster by directly typing in your findings or dragging and dropping figures. Be cognizant of font size—most readers of your poster will stand 3 to 6 feet away, so make sure your font is significantly large to be read; typically, 24 to 36 point is adequate for the text of the poster. Once you have the poster completed, it will have to be printed, which will have a cost associated with it. Your institution may have an internal source for printing or may provide you with templates to use—it may also cover the cost of printing. Keep your poster as uncluttered as possible in areas like the abstract, introduction, and conclusion, using brief text in these areas. Use of tables, infographics, and figures is appropriate in the methods and results sections, but have sufficient text so that your reader can easily follow the rationale for the project, how it was done, and the outcomes. Posters are read from left to right, top to bottom, like pages of a book, so make sure the flow of your poster feels natural to the reader. Finally, posters are most often printed on either paper or fabric. For a paper poster, make sure you have a sturdy cardboard tube for the poster to protect it as you travel to a conference. There are commercially available plastic poster tubes that come equipped with straps and are adjustable. If you find yourself presenting posters often, they may be worth purchasing as they make onboard carrying and travel much easier. Fabric posters are often more convenient for travel as they may be folded and easily stored. For either medium, if you are traveling to your conference, make sure your poster is in your carry-on materials so that it arrives at your presentation along with you. Note that some larger conference venues may also have options for electronic poster formats. In instances like these, you will upload your poster to a database and then it will be available to you on a screen at your designated poster time. There might also be an option for you to record audio to give a viewer a "walk through" of your poster in a self-guided way. If an electronic poster is an option, make certain to read the details for submission carefully so that your poster is visible to viewers without any issues.

## Oral Presentations

If you are giving an oral presentation, you may need to submit your slides well in advance of your talk, so it is a good idea to have the project at a point where data collection is either completed or near completion. Do not submit slides that are conjectures of results. As you prepare to present, it is vital that you pay attention to time allotted for the presentation. Your abstract may have been accepted for a 15- or 30-minute oral presentation. If you are accustomed to presenting your findings in a longer (or shorter) time frame, you will have to adapt your slides. If you need to fill a bit of time, it is always good to include evidence at the start of the talk. This will set the rationale for your project and will familiarize those in the audience who may not have a grasp on your area of expertise. Then, follow with slides on methods and results. Your presentation should leave time for questions at the end. One last note, if you are co-presenting with a colleague, make sure the transitions between you are logical and seamless. Practice the transitions in advance, as well as who will begin and end the session. In all, practice does indeed make perfect. Practicing your session will let you know how much time it will take, where you may need to add or subtract content, and will familiarize you with content that may be challenging (e.g., drug or condition nomenclature, explanations of statistics).

### Oral Presentation Guidelines

As you consider preparing your oral presentation, you may be tempted to squeeze as much detail onto each slide so that you don't forget to share everything with the audience. However, it is important to remember that just like a poster will not convey the level of complexity and detail that your work represents, neither will the slides for your presentation. Rather, think of the slides as a mechanism to provide your audience with an outline of your talk to make it easier for them to follow along. Consider following the 10-20-30 rule of PowerPoint (Microsoft; Kawasaki, n.d.). This rule advocates that based on an audience's attention and your ability to captivate them, you present 10 slides during a talk that lasts no more than 20 minutes and uses a font that is no smaller than 30 points. You might find yourself tinkering

with this formula, but the point is that less is better. It is also a visual stimulus that can help clarify any complex concepts you mention or can be used to share a visual representation of a scenario or equipment you might be discussing. There are a number of excellent resources available online for free (Design Shack, 2010; GCFGlobal, n.d.).

Keep your slides clean—not over-cluttered with pictures, graphs, and tables. Consider how inclusive and accessible your materials are, particularly in virtual presentations (Hernandez et al., 2022). Remember, if you are presenting in a large room, those at the back of the room should be able to see clearly what is on the slides. Consider using fonts that are no smaller than 30 points for your text, and larger fonts should be used for slide titles. Use an easily legible font (e.g., Arial, Times New Roman), and make sure there is sufficient contrast between text and your slide background. Use bullet points rather than complete sentences, and if you are using borrowed figures, artwork, or data, make sure you have permission for use and acknowledge the use (typically in the Notes section of the slide). For a poster, make sure your text is legible from 3 to 6 feet away. Your participant should not have to stand at the poster to read salient points; doing so will obstruct the view for other interested attendees.

To ensure your presentation goes well, you must practice it! A good suggestion is to go through the talk uninterrupted at least three times. It may take you several attempts before you can do this as you may find that certain slides are too simple, too complex, or add little value to the presentation. Changes to your talk are best made well before you practice it for presentation. If you find that changes must be made near your presentation time, the changes should not be substantive. Most often, time can be "found" in the early part of the talk. For instance, you may have opted to include a slide on the different types of stroke and how they present in the affected patient. In the interest of time, you may tell your audience "Slide 4 in your handout details information on the pathology included in this talk" and move on. It is more expeditious to spend time on results, discussion, and questions than background, but the best talk will have a balance of all components. This is why rehearsal is so important!

---

## Box 11-1:
## Presenting and Feedback Cycle

Your board of mentors can serve many roles as you think about presenting your work. Consider soliciting help with proofreading conference submissions, as well as slides and posters. Board members could also listen to you practice a talk and provide you with valuable feedback.

Figure 11-1 shows an example of a slide deck with recommended fonts for your presentation. As you create your presentation, remember to use a high-contrast background and font. PowerPoint (or whatever software you choose) has free infographics that may be used in presentations. These are under the Insert tab on the PowerPoint toolbar. Infographics add visual appeal to the presentation while making major points clear to the participant. The example shows a few infographics. If you use figures, pictures, diagrams, or video clips in your presentation, make sure you cite their source and include permissions for use, and make sure that they will work if you need to use different equipment at the speaking venue. The sample slide deck includes how to cite figures used in a presentation.

## Putting a Presentation Together

All presentations consist of similar components: a title page with author affiliations; a slide discussing any conflicts of interest you may have or research sponsorships; a slide with learning objectives for your audience; background information that supports your hypothesis; results to date; discussion of results, including relevance to your field and limitations of the study; future directions; and references. If you are presenting a poster, you will also provide an abstract defining the project. Each of these are briefly discussed next.

### Title and Conflict of Interest Slides

While it may seem obvious, the first slide should state the title of your presentation, your name, credentials, and your affiliation. If the project had contributors who are not presenting, all should be listed either here or on a subsequent slide with credentials. Do not leave off authors of the work if you are presenting solo. All contributors should get credit for the presentation, whether they are on the stage or not. Your conflict(s) of interest will list any financial or personal relationships that could influence the data. This may include funding sources, sponsorships, or your personal use of a product or service described in the presentation. For posters, the title and authors will run across the top of the poster.

### Abstract and/or Objectives

If you are presenting a poster, you will include a short abstract of your work as the first block of the poster. An abstract is a brief (typically between 100 to 500 words) description of your hypothesis with a bit of relevant context, your methods, your results, and a sentence or two of discussion. In an oral presentation, typically the abstract is not included on a slide. Here, after the title slide, a slide of learning objectives

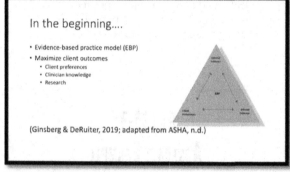

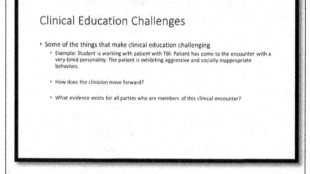

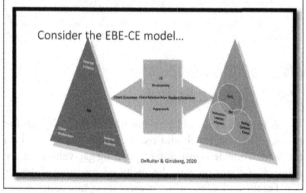

**Figure 11-1.** Obtaining feedback.

will be shown. These are vetted by the organization for whom you are presenting to make sure they meet the scientific rigor, needs, interests, and acumen of the audience. When writing objectives, use higher order words from Bloom's taxonomy, such as "categorize," "classify," "appraise," "examine," and "choose" in each objective. Some examples follow.

## Box 11-2:
### Sample Learning Objectives

Following this presentation, the learner will:

1. List a range of options for familiarizing graduate students in speech-language pathology with new patients.

2. Appraise different methods of patient familiarization in a speech-language pathology university clinic.

3. Identify and choose strategies for familiarizing graduate students in speech-language pathology with new patients on their caseload.

## Box 11-3:
### Abstract Example

Graduate students in university speech-language pathology clinics may have a variety of options for familiarizing themselves with new patients on their caseloads. One option may be video recordings of goal-directed patient performance during therapy. This study examined graduate student preferences for viewing a recording from an entire session 1 week before the new graduate clinician was responsible for the case vs. a "highlight reel" of performance on various goals across multiple sessions in a 4-week time span. Analysis of results indicated a preference for a "highlight reel" with novice clinicians reporting they were able to glean more goal-specific information regarding patient performance (adapted from DeRuiter & Hinderscheit, 2009).

## Background Information Supporting Your Project

A few slides should be dedicated to the "why" of the project. These slides should recall current or past work in the field, while demonstrating a learning gap validating the research. References may be included on these slides or listed at the end. For a poster presentation, this panel would be called "Introduction." Depending on the length of the oral talk, you may choose to go into detail in this section. If you have limited time (15 minutes), this section may be a slide or two, but it must be included to set the stage for your methods, results, and discussion.

## Methods, Results, and Discussion Slides

These slides are the "meat" of your presentation—they are what have drawn audience members to your talk, so it is essential to flesh out your process and results. The methods should be specific enough for the audience member to understand the process. An adage in research science is that the learner should be able to exactly replicate the work based on your methods. While this holds true for peer-reviewed publications in scientific journals, for presentation, it is often sufficient to present the main facets of your experiment: number of subjects, equipment or tools used, statistical methods used, and any parameters of the study that define your methods (e.g., "adults 18 and older were included," "only children who were receiving home-based services for speech were included"). Often, methods are presented in two to three slides. On a poster, methods are in their own panel labeled "Methods."

Results are presented in a variety of ways. You may opt to use a table of results (depending on statistical methods) with significant results marked with a symbol, such as an asterisk. Unless it affects your study, data that was not statistically significant, although presented, may be something that you opt not to discuss in a short time frame. Your discussion of results should encompass significant findings that are relevant for your audience. If time permits, nonstatistically significant data or other interesting facets of the study may be discussed. In the earlier example of objectives, one of them was to "appraise different methods of reducing anxiety in undergraduate nursing students as they transition to acute-care clinical environments across semesters." If your results demonstrate that those students receiving specific classroom instruction in nuances of their new environment show significant decreases in anxiety, while web-based asynchronous lectures that reviewed general nursing content and general advising support sessions were all similar and less effective, spend time on the significant part of your results. This will also help form your discussion. The discussion should not be a reiteration of the results, rather it should help the learner interpret the results. In the previous example, it may inform health care educators that the least effective tool for reducing anxiety in undergraduate nursing students who are transitioning to acute-care environments is general advising support. This may inform clinical decisions. Does it? Unless you have evidence to prove that it does, your discussion ends with informing the learner of possibilities. Explain to your audience what your results mean in the context of evidence found in the literature associated with the discipline. In other words, this is not a time to proffer opinions or "curbside" consults. Consider the presentation an opportunity to educate your audience on a topic in which you are honing expertise. A future study might focus on how this issue fits with other

# Box 11-4:
## Quick Tips for Presenting Your Findings

The venue at which you present your research may vary from a small, institution-based facility (with an audience of 10 or less) to a major national or international conference with potentially hundreds of attendees. The following are tips for all presentations, no matter the size or scope of the audience.

1. Practice, practice, practice. If you are giving an oral presentation, practice out loud so that you know how the presentation will flow and how long the presentation will take. Often, when presenting in front of an audience, one tends to speak a bit faster, so keep this in mind as you practice staying within your time constraints. If you are presenting with a colleague, practice together so that transitions are seamless, and you know how much time each of you will have for the presentation.

2. Know your audience. Recognize that you may have students, allied health professionals, and colleagues in the audience; make sure the level of presentation is suitable for most of the audience.

3. Introduce yourself if the moderator of your presentation has not done so. Acknowledge the moderator if they have introduced you.

4. Dress appropriately.

5. Speak with confidence. You are the content expert of your presentation!

6. Use figures to illustrate points and augment your slides, but remember, you may need to acquire permission to use figures and artwork in your talk.

7. Keep slides (or your poster) as "clean" as possible. Fewer words, not jumbled with figures. Use bullet points. Do not use complete sentences. Spend no more than 1 to 2 minutes per slide.

8. Practice using the technology, including the microphone and the slide advancer. If you are presenting virtually, familiarize yourself with the platform in use, including sound and volume controls.

9. Acknowledge questions. Depending on your audience and venue, questions may be encouraged throughout your presentation or held to the end. Do not get so involved in a reply that you cannot present your results and discussion.

10. If you are presenting a poster, be at the poster for the entire slotted time. If you are absent, meeting attendees will not have the opportunity to engage with you. Install and remove your poster within the guidelines you are given by the meeting organizers.

elements of nursing education. A good ending for an oral or poster presentation is to show that you have considered the significance of your findings and where they might lead. A "Future Directions" slide following the discussion shows the learner that you are interested in pursuing this path of research because it may have relevance to practice.

## References and Questions

Make sure to include a slide (or more) of relevant references at the end of your talk. Your conference organizer will instruct you of the format of references (e.g., American Psychological Association, Chicago Manual of Style). An up-to-date reference list allows learners to investigate the topic further, using references you used to frame and test your hypothesis. There is no need to linger on this slide or discuss it in the presentation. Rather, move on to a final slide that asks audience members if they have questions regarding any aspect of the talk. Remember, the objectives

you presented should be measurable and clear. You will quickly learn from questions directed to you whether your presentation met its stated objectives. If there is a lack of understanding, it is perfectly acceptable to use this time to further explain a concept that participants found to be murky. Often, questions spark something you may not have considered, and this may shape future research on your project. Rarely, there will be no questions following a presentation. Since you have allotted time for questions, use this time to engage your audience with a question of your own. An example might include soliciting audience participants to share an experience with the topic you are presenting. A general question, such as "Would anyone care to share an experience they have had with medication administration in stroke patients?," may spark discussion. At times, questioners may express disagreement with your research premise or conclusions. View these questions as an opportunity to both educate and expand your professional growth. Actively listen to questions—repeating them for clarity and for the benefit of all attendees. Use a positive tone and body language, and if you are stumped by a question, it is far more professional to admit a lack of knowledge than to ignore the question or manufacture an answer. Most oral presentation sessions have a moderator who will suggest that further questioning may occur after the session, so make yourself available. Do not infringe on the allotted time of the next presenter by continuing to engage in discussion in excess of your session. Professional audiences may be very engaged; they are rarely antagonistic in their questioning, and your expertise and passion for your research will set a positive tone.

## Virtual Versus Live Presentations: Increasing Engagement and Active Listening

If your conference is virtual, the same tips and "rules" of presenting apply, with a few caveats. First, make sure you are familiar with all technology the conference host is using. If you are anxious about it, most organizers will allow you to meet with technical staff to help you prior to your presentation. Timing is important in the virtual world—make sure your presentation fits the parameters, leaving time for questions. Use a professional or blurred background so that it is not distracting to viewers. Remember to look into your computer camera, or on screen, and not at the thumbnail of yourself as you present (if it is visible). If your internet connection is unstable, acknowledge that and repeat key points learners may have missed. Better, use a hotspot or reliable technology when you present.

## Asynchronous Versus Synchronous Presentations

Most oral presentations at conferences will be in the synchronous format, which means that you will present your talk in real time to an audience of live listeners. On the day of your talk or poster, make sure you arrive at the venue early. If you are presenting a poster, this will allow you to see where you will be, and whether there are supplies (e.g., tacks, pins) provided for your use. In the case of an oral presentation, arriving early will let you gauge the audience size, the lighting, temperature, and acoustics of the room. Although most conferences adhere closely to published times, the presenter prior to you may finish a bit early (or late). Typically, there will be sufficient time between talks for you to quickly check that your slides, the microphone, the pointer, and any other equipment you may need is functioning. At most conferences, there is a technical support person to help should anything go wrong.

## ACTIVE LISTENING AND PARTICIPANT ENGAGEMENT

We have discussed types of audiences and tips for presenting synchronously in depth, but your invitation to present may be in an asynchronous format—meaning, you will likely record your talk and participants will be given a link to access it. Synchronous presentations allow for audience interaction, lively question and answer periods, and even debate. Asynchronous presentations may feel a bit sterile in contrast. But there are effective ways to make both synchronous and asynchronous presentations engaging. Keeping your time constraints in mind, add a few slides that cause your participant to think about the problem you are discussing and possible ways to solve it. Typically, a question slide inserted early into the talk will start the process of learner engagement. You may decide to give the "answer" to the question slide in a subsequent slide, or hold it until later in the talk. Highlight the correct answer so that attendees can read it for understanding. Placing questions in a talk is a good way to involve listeners in a process of understanding your hypothesis and making sense of your results. Make sure your questions are in alignment with the objectives of your talk. An example question using our earlier objectives follows:

---

### Box 11-5:
### Sample Slide Question

Students who demonstrate challenges in health care documentation typically exhibit?

A.  A tendency to procrastinate

B.  Poor writing abilities across the board

C.  Time management challenges in the clinical environment

D.  None of the above

---

Typically, wait no more than 10 to 15 seconds after proposing your question to move on; the learner will see it again when you post the answer. For a 15- to 30-minute talk, three to five questions should be included to ensure active learning and engagement. When attendees have an active role in the presentation, their retention and understanding of the information will be enhanced.

Following a conference presentation, you may receive notification of learner feedback from your talk. Attendees are often asked to provide impressions of the presentation with respect to content and learning outcomes. Understand that even the best presentation will have its detractors, so do not be disappointed if the feedback is not completely positive. Utilize the ratings and comments received to better hone your content and presentation style.

## Box 11-6:
## Hybrid Presentations

Some conference options might be truly hybrid. You might upload a prerecorded presentation for viewers to review during a multi-day period. Then, you might find a conference organizer asks you to be available for a question-and-answer segment during a very specific time period. This segment might be one where you answer questions over a video format or via webchat.

## Conclusion

Sharing your research findings at a conference of any size is an exciting opportunity for professional growth. Developing expertise in presenting takes diligence, practice, organization, and skill, but presenting tends to get easier each time you do it. Dissemination of research findings is the necessary outcome of the scientific method, and you will find that sharing knowledge with your colleagues at professional conferences will become an enriching part of your career.

## References

DeRuiter, M., & Hinderscheit, L. (2009). Preparing student clinicians: Comparing video composites to full-session recordings. Poster presentation at the Annual Convention of the American Speech-Language-Hearing Association, New Orleans, LA.

Design Shack. (2010). *10 tips for designing presentations that don't suck: Part 2.* https://designshack.net/articles/graphics/10-tips-for-designing-presentations-that-don%E2%80%99t-suck-pt-2/

GCFGlobal. (n.d.). *Simple rules for better PowerPoint presentations.* https://edu.gcfglobal.org/en/powerpoint-tips/simple-rules-for-better-powerpoint-presentations/1/

Hernandez, L. A., Chodkowski, N., & Treibergs, K. (2022). A guide to implementing inclusive and accessible virtual poster sessions. *Journal of Microbiology and Biology Education,* 23(1), e00237-21. https://www.ncbi.nlm.nih.gov/pmc/articles/PMC9053039/

Kawasaki, G. (n.d.). *The 10/20/30 rule of PowerPoint.* https://guykawasaki.com/the_102030_rule/

New York University. (2022, July 20). *How to create a research poster.* https://guides.nyu.edu/posters

Pinch, E. (2022, June 7). *How to create beautiful and effective academic posters in PowerPoint.* BrightCarbon. https://www.brightcarbon.com/blog/effective-academic-posters-powerpoint/

# Worksheet 11-1:
# Presenting Your Research

What is the focus of your research presentation?

Who is your audience?

**Presentation Venues**

| State and Local | National and International |
|---|---|
| Plan A: | Plan A: |
| Plan B: | Plan B: |

Presentation format preferences: poster or oral?

*(continued)*

# Worksheet 11-1:
# Presenting Your Research (continued)

**Presentation Outline**

- Disclosures/conflicts of interest
- Acknowledge funding (if applicable)
- Background information (why?)
- Methods
- Results
- Discussion
- References (key/select list)
- Questions (question-and-answer time)

Presentation strategies: How can you increase audience active engagement?

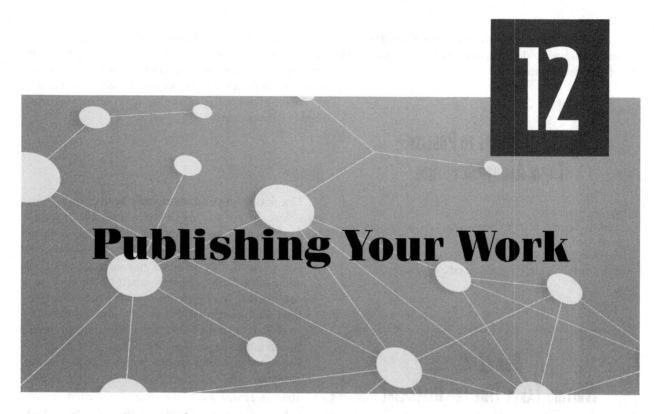

# Publishing Your Work

*Mark DeRuiter, MBA, PhD, CCC-A/SLP, F-ASHA*
*and Sarah M. Ginsberg, EdD, CCC-SLP, F-ASHA*

If you take yourself back to Chapter 2 of this text, you'll recall that we discussed backward design and a quote from Stephen Covey (1989):

> To begin with the end in mind means to start with a clear understanding of your destination. It means to know where you're going so that you better understand where you are now so that the steps you take are always in the right direction.
> —Stephen Covey, *The Seven Habits of Highly Effective People*

This chapter is designed to get you thinking about publishing your work and what it will take to be successful in that process. There is no "magic bullet" for publishing, and it isn't necessarily easy work. Instead, you will be required to put forth your best manuscript and typically have it reviewed by your peers. This means that what you initially submit and what is finally published might look like reasonably different pieces of work. This is a good thing because you have had the opportunity to incorporate what we call "the gift of feedback" into your process. But it takes time, discipline, and energy! This is why there can be a significant lag in the time it takes you to complete your work and see it in print. However, if you start with a specific end in mind, you may be able to adapt your work and timelines accordingly.

## TIME FOR REFLECTION

Take a moment to reflect on the questions you would like to answer, how you might conduct your research, and where you would like to publish your work. If you don't have an immediate answer to the "where," think through these questions:

- Who do you want to talk to, and where will you find your audience?

- Is the question you are answering in your research important to that audience?

- Is it something you will publish in a book? A journal? Will it be a research note? Part of a newsletter? A web page? A blog?

DeRuiter, M., & Ginsberg, S. M. (Eds.). *Clinician's Guide to Applying, Conducting, and Disseminating Clinical Education Research* (pp. 145-156).
© 2024 Taylor & Francis Group.

Give yourself some time to think about your ideal final product right now and make some notes on the work and where it might be published.

---

### Box 12-1: Where to Publish—Think About the Future

It's important to consider where to publish. For instance, publishers are going to want to know if your work has been published elsewhere and you are going to need to make an attestation whether or not the work has been previously disseminated. Publishing in a blog might feel like a "quick win" but be problematic later.

---

### Box 12-2: Writing Takes Time and Discipline

You'll want to block off time for writing, just like you might set aside time for exercise or meditating. The point is, writing takes time (Quinn & Rush, 2009). Mark finds that he needs to be "in the mood" to write. He's found that can make for an easy excuse *not* to write. However, Mark has found there can be activities to get him ready to write—a little chocolate, coffee, and sometimes a beautiful view can help! Sarah's strategy is scheduling time to write and sticking to that schedule. She can find ways to "hide away" and write by closing up email and limiting other distractions. In the end, you need to do what works for you, and talking with peers and your board of mentors can be helpful. Take in all kinds of suggestions and allow yourself to be curious and try a few different options. It can take a little time to figure out the best strategy for you, but it can have a great payoff.

---

There are lots of terms and things to think about when it comes to publishing. We've put together Table 12-1 for you to use as you think through some of these basic pieces of information. You might want to refer to it now and as you move throughout this chapter.

## Where to Publish

Although it's not possible to advise you on exactly where to publish your work, we can walk you through the range of common options. We'll discuss some of the high points, and some of the challenges along the way. Note that we'll spend a fair amount of time discussing journal articles. This is mainly due to the fact that this might be one area that has the most access for you. For now, take a look at this range of options as you reflect upon where your work might be disseminated.

## Books

One option for publication might be that you are writing a book chapter or even an entire book. The important thing to remember here is that writing for books is a contractual process that typically begins one of two ways:

- You are invited by an editor to contribute to a book and contractually obligate yourself to the work. In a case like this, you might be invited to write a chapter or more for a given book. You are typically invited directly by the editor of the book themselves, and you should be seeking guidance from them about what they want you to write in your chapter with a potential outline of topics.

- You engage with a publisher/acquisitions editor to publish an entire book on your own (as a sole author or author/editor). Note that it won't be as simple as this. A publisher will likely require you to submit a book prospectus where you discuss the need for the book, how your book will meet that need, and even chapter outlines. It is possible that the publisher will send your prospectus out to peers to determine the viability and necessity of your proposal. It's also possible that the acquisitions editor will come back to you with specific thoughts and edits that you will have to weigh before you make a decision regarding the contract and the process.

If you will serve as the editor for a book, you might contribute your own work and invite colleagues who are experts in their areas to contribute as well (much like the workbook you are reading!). You might find that you need to reach out to find these experts, and here is where your board of mentors (Chapter 5) could be very helpful to you.

Regardless, books will require contracts for publishing. In the world of book publishing you will want to consider whether the published book is available by print, electronically, or both. You'll also want to consider issues related to payment and royalties, which go beyond the scope of this chapter. However, if you publish a book/publish a chapter in a book, note that you will typically assign copyright to the publisher meaning that they hold the rights to the content, and you are agreeing not to publish the work elsewhere.

Book publishers will have editors and editorial teams. However, the review process of your work may not be as rigorous as what you might find should you elect to submit original research to a peer-reviewed journal. There also isn't

*Table 12-1*

# Basic Terms in Publishing

| TERM | MEANING |
|---|---|
| Author | The author is the person writing the work. This will be you! However, there could be multiple authors of a manuscript. |
| Manuscript | This is the draft of your work. Usually, a manuscript will be written to specifications indicated by the publisher. |
| Publisher | The entity that disseminates your work (often a company). |
| Editor | The person who edits your work for publication. |
| Acquisitions editor | An editor who has a primary responsibility to bring authors and their work to a publisher. |
| Reviewer | Often a peer who has content knowledge who reviews and edits your work for content, rigor, design, and other edits. |
| Copyright | A term for intellectual property and the right for a person or organization to distribute, display, and even adapt this property for a period of time. |
| Double-blind reviews | Reviews where the authors' and reviewers' identities are not shared. |
| Copyeditor | Editor who reviews manuscripts immediately before publication to make certain all final elements of the document are in order. |
| Page proofs/galley proofs | A final version of your document for review, immediately before it is published. This would be your "last chance" to make any small changes to your work before it is published. |
| e-books | Books that are published online. |
| Paywall | In online venues, the point where a reader must pay/login to gain access to a certain work. |
| Open access | Dissemination venues where readers do not encounter a paywall. Free login accounts may be required. |

necessarily an exact outline that you will follow for writing up your work. Instead, you may have an editor propose an outline or structure to you, or creating the structure of an outline will be your role as author/editor. Consistent chapter outlines can be what gives an academic textbook a look and feel of consistency across chapters. It is worth noting that while journal articles will often have more of a predictable outline, books will be something negotiated and typically more open. Considering the outline is what can be very stimulating for some writers—you might prefer something more formulaic (like journal articles) or creative (like books).

Books are a great way for you to disseminate your work. However, this can feel challenging and less accessible for some authors, especially if your work is not well-known. This is due to the fact that you might not know the right people who will invite you, or you don't have connections with a publisher. Give yourself time for your career to grow! The publication of smaller works is a great way to get noticed and move forward with chapters and books. However, the aforementioned reasons are why other venues or journal articles are often a first choice.

## Box 12-3:
## Book Timelines

One large consideration with books (whether for a chapter or an entire book) is the contractual obligation. You are setting yourself to complete work that often will have a defined number of pages, tables and figures, and timelines. Timelines are often the biggest challenge for authors. It's important to think about your lifestyle, work, and critical events as you make a commitment to a timeline. Additionally, you need to stay on task and write regularly to keep yourself motivated to complete the manuscript on time. If you believe you are running into problems that might pose delays, you should be connecting with your publisher early to let them know about your challenges and your plan for mitigating them.

# Other Venues

## State- or Regional-Level Professional Organization Publications

There could be a variety of options to consider with some basic internet searching. For instance, there could be state- or regional-level publication opportunities to disseminate your work to readers who are members of organizations. These might be an excellent way to move some of your work forward with editorial review that is less rigorous than what we will describe for journal articles. In this case, remember that you might be limiting your work to readers who are members of a particular group or association, particularly if your work will require a login for access (in online environments, others outside of the organization may encounter a paywall where they would be required to pay to gain access to the work). Sometimes opportunities to publish in these venues might come to you as you present your work (see Chapter 11). It is possible that a conference attendee or coordinator might make you aware of a publication opportunity. Listen carefully regarding any options, but don't immediately commit until you have had a chance to explore the exact nature of what is being proposed to you. This way you can verify that the work you might publish will reach your intended audience.

## Institutional Publications

Another option might be for research that is site- or institution-specific. For instance, some university or health care settings will have options for publication of materials on their websites or through newsletters. As with the previously mentioned options, these types of publications are likely edited but not critically reviewed. Note that some organizational newsletters might also have a related web page or other form of electronic publication that is easily accessible to your peers. Although, this is not always a guarantee. If you are entirely new to the publication process, this could be a reasonable start for you; just make certain of the accessibility of your work to your intended audience.

## Blogs

We've already mentioned blogs. This can be a creative way to write about your work (and yourself!). We have already cautioned you to consider what you "give away" in a blog— because it can be considered a form of publication, which you would need to disclose in the future. However, blogs can be a way for you to develop a "following" for you and your work. An additional way to use a blog might be to write more about the theoretical aspects of your work and avoid publishing results. This would give you the opportunity to publish the actual data in another venue down the road. It might also give you an opportunity to gather feedback from readers that could contribute to improving your work in advance of data publication, as part of the feedback process mentioned in Chapter 10.

# Journals

We've left journals for last, and we certainly hope you will consider them. There can be some advantages to publishing in journals that can include access and prestige. That said, publishing in journals can also be a bit challenging in terms of understanding the process. We'll talk more about these in this section and work to give you tips for publishing in this type of venue. Keep in mind, some of these tips might be useful to you regardless of where you publish!

When you are conducting research, collecting data, and assimilating your findings, it is important to consider the rigor of your work. Rigor refers to how the experimentation is done—does the research answer important questions in the discipline? Did you seek institutional review board approval for the projects? These things are covered earlier in this text. If your data stand the tests of academic rigor, you may want to submit a manuscript to a peer-reviewed journal. We've mentioned peer review before, and we'll talk more deeply about what "peer reviewed" means in a moment.

To share your information with a broader audience, you might want to consider publishing in a journal that is open-access and national or international. There are several choices to choose from, but the "safe choice" is one that is affiliated with your profession or organization. If there is a journal that you are considering publishing in, but you are not confident that your research would be accepted by the journal, it may be helpful to reach out to the journal's editor and inquire, explaining very briefly the nature of your study. You can also consult a section on the journal's web pages that are likely to be labeled "Aims and Scope" that are intended to indicate what type of work the journal is focused on publishing. This will help you further decide if the journal is a good fit for your work. When you submit your manuscript to a peer-reviewed journal, it is typically given a high-level review by the journal editor(s) first. At this point, the editor may accept or reject your article as potentially suitable for the journal. If accepted for review, it will be sent to scholars in the area of your expertise. Peer review is typically conducted "double-blind"—meaning, you will not know the reviewer's identity, and they will not know yours. This allows for an unbiased review of the work. The most prestigious, trusted journals rely on the peer-review process to ensure that published work is novel, meets the standards of academic rigor, and will significantly add to knowledge in the field.

## Box 12-4: Acceptance Rates and Publishing Strategies

A major consideration will be the odds of whether your article will be published in a journal (or not!). We've mentioned reaching out to editors, and it might be worth asking an editor if they can tell you the percentage of manuscripts submitted that are actually accepted and published. Often "more prestigious" journals will have a lower acceptance rate. You'll want to think about this very carefully. How much time are you willing to wait to get an answer from a prestigious journal in your field? Would it be better for you to begin your path with publishing in a venue that is lower in status to get your work in front of your audience? Would the feedback from the highly acclaimed journal be invaluable? We cannot answer these questions for you. However, having information as you consider your options can be very helpful. Also, make sure to lean on your board of mentors who may be more experienced in this area!

An alternative journal choice is to publish in a scholarship of teaching and learning (SoTL) journal. This is not a less safe choice but submitting to this type of journal will take some thoughtful writing on your part. When you are writing for a journal that is connected to your own field, the relevance of the problem, and even much of the vocabulary, is familiar to your audience, the readers. However, when you submit your work to a SoTL journal, you must make small modifications that move the focus of your work from the specific context that you conducted the study in and identify how it can broadly be of value to readers from other related fields looking to identify evidence-based education-clinical education practices. Explain how the problem that you were looking to learn about is important not just to your specific discipline but to any clinical educator working with novice clinicians in health-related fields. The goal with these journals is to help the readers understand the context, including the challenges and opportunities, that exist in the setting that you are teaching in so that others can draw on the information and make connections to the clinical education work they are doing in their discipline and their setting (Bernstein, 2011). Explain aspects of the teaching and learning more explicitly than you would if you were writing for your discipline in particular. The advantage of submitting your manuscript to a SoTL journal is that you reach a broader audience, one that goes beyond the confines of your discipline and can initiate learning and discussion that benefits a wider group of readers.

## Overview of the Peer-Review Process

One thing to consider when you want to publish your work is the peer-review process. In a few words, here is how peer review works:

- An editor is assigned to your work. Typically, this is someone who has expertise in the content area where you are publishing. However, it is not always guaranteed your editor will have deep content knowledge of your area.
- The editor works with a team of peer reviewers who take your work and critically evaluate it. This process can take weeks to months. A few of the broad elements that reviewers are looking for:
  - The importance of your work in the context of your content area
  - Scientific rigor
  - Clarity of the work
  - Soundness of the methods you used to answer your questions
  - How well you acknowledge the broader context of your work both historically and in the future

Peer review typically is viewed as the "highest level" of publication. The process is not trivial, and we will discuss the outcomes more in the following section. What is important to note is that choosing where your work is published is part of beginning with the end in mind: Do you have professional or personal goals regarding where your work is published and how it is viewed by your colleagues? This can become very important in academic circles where quality of peer-reviewed work might mean more than multiple non–peer-reviewed publications. In order to aid your thinking, Figure 12-1 gives you a sense of the continuum of publications and the review process.

### Peer Review: Timelines, Decisions, and Communications

Recognize that the peer-review process takes time; once you submit an article to an editor at a journal, it may take months before you will hear back from the journal. Most journals use electronic platforms where you can do some general tracking of your manuscript along the way. The journal's website may also tell you the expected time frame. However, not many details can be shared with you to ensure the double-blind process.

As previously mentioned, typically your work will be reviewed by a minimum of two reviewers, and these reviews are synthesized by an editor who will respond with a decision about the manuscript. Notifications regarding your paper will come in several forms: accepted with no revisions, accepted with (minor or major) revisions, or rejected. It is rare for a manuscript to be accepted with no revisions. Requested revisions may be as minor as editorial

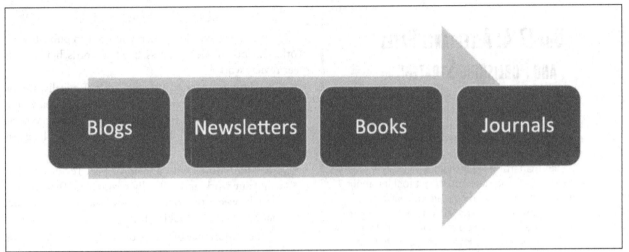

**Figure 12-1.** Broad publication categories listed by rigor of review (from no review on the left to rigorous review on the right).

and grammatical changes or as major as requesting additional experimentation and evidence. Make sure you adhere to deadlines that editors will set for all changes to be made. If for some reason you are challenged to meet the editor's deadline, reach out and discuss the possibility of an extension. Note the editor is not obligated to offer you an extension, so clear and polite communication will be valuable in obtaining your desired result.

You must consider and answer all reviewer comments, even if you find the comments "unfair" or having missed the point. Note that just because a reviewer suggests a change, you do not have to make the change. If you decide against making a suggested change, your rationale should be explained in your response to the reviewers. Be professional in your answers to reviewers; if it is necessary to refute comments, provide evidence. You may also have to decide whether it is feasible and expedient to make requested revisions. If additional experimentation is called for and you no longer have access to a specific patient or student clinician population, for instance, it is likely that additional evidence cannot be provided to make the manuscript acceptable. Do not despair! This is not necessarily the end of your data dissemination. Perhaps a different journal or a different format might be a strategy to pursue.

## Box 12-5:
## Reading Between the Lines

The peer-review process is long. It might be tempting to consider submitting your work to multiple journals at once. This is not advised. In most instances, you are making a clear commitment to an editor and publisher that your work is not being considered elsewhere and *only* in the journal where you have submitted it.

Occasionally, you might receive a response from an editor that feels rather unclear. For instance, the editor might indicate that you are welcome to "resubmit the work after you have reviewed the reviewer comments" or you might be told, "This work is not a fit for our journal at this time." Bluntly put, these are kind ways of rejecting your work. If you plan to resubmit the work, you should have a conversation with the editor about the reality of acceptance to the journal vs. spending many hours trying to adjust a manuscript to fit a vague promise. Often, these kind messages are ways of indicating to you to "look elsewhere."

## Box 12-6:
## Edited Versus Peer Reviewed

Disambiguating "peer reviewed" from "edited" can be helpful as you consider disseminating your work. Think of it this way: *Edited works* are reviewed by editors for their content (broadly) and clarity. An editor might have suggestions for you to make sure that your work is "consumable" by the proposed audience, and they may have grammatical and organizational suggestions. The best outcome is when your editor also has content knowledge. In this case, they can also provide feedback on your content. *Peer-reviewed works* will go one layer deeper. Along with editorial comments, peer reviewers will be looking closely at the rigor of your research (e.g., how it was designed, how it contributes to your discipline both now and in the future), and they will make editorial suggestions as well. Peer review is often considered the highest level of review.

## Writing Up Your Work for a Journal: The Manuscript

If a journal is your choice, where do you begin? The first thing you will want to do is outline your work. The document you will produce will be called a *manuscript*. Consider it your draft of the work you are submitting to an editor and peer-review team (possibly) at a journal or other publisher. It might sound trivial, but working from an outline can be useful to you in a variety of ways:

- It helps you break the work into manageable pieces (especially when your time is limited for writing).

- You'll be able to conceptualize some areas and write them with less effort and get them moving forward ahead of time (e.g., background and methods; we will discuss this more subsequently). This can give you a feeling of accomplishment and inspire you to keep going.

- You'll be able to understand the logical flow of your "story" and how you will guide the reader through each element if you start with an outline.

### Article Structure

Odds are you examined other research before you started on your own. We've talked about that throughout this workbook, and particularly in Chapters 4 and 8. Never underestimate the power of adhering to a structure of what you have seen in the places where you aspire your work to be published. For instance, if you are looking for a submission to a peer-reviewed journal, you will likely find this type of order to the outline of the work:

- Title: The title of your work should give readers a clear indication of what your publication is about. Note that some journals will have word or character limits relative to the title. A good title will capture the attention of your intended audience without making any exaggerated claims. Make sure to verify with the journal instructions about the use of acronyms in any journal titles. You might need to spell out every word, even with common acronyms.

- Abstract: This is a short summary of your work. It will briefly cover the necessity for the research, what you found, and why the findings are important. It's easiest to write this last.

- Introduction/Background: Here you are setting the stage for the identified research question and what we know/do not know about it. You'll be able to start on this relatively early because it is the core set of reasons for why you have conceptualized the overall work. Sometimes writing this section can reveal to you where existing "holes" are in your thinking. It is important to clear these up as quickly as possible so that your research is based upon a sound review of the literature.

- Research Question: This should be apparent to you before even getting going! You'll want to make the question clear to your reader so there are no assumptions. If you are wondering what to title your manuscript, looking at the research question can be a great start.

- Hypotheses: If you are conducting quantitative work, you will likely have hypotheses. These will be developed early in your process and something you can commit to writing easily, once you have established them. These will be closely linked to your research question and involve what you are specifically testing. If your work is qualitative in nature, you will not have specific hypotheses per se. You might have ideas about what you might anticipate finding, but these will not be stated in qualitative research manuscripts.

- Methods: In this section, you will report what a reader needs to know in order to replicate your work. You'll want to keep detailed notes of your work and the process you engaged in for your research. Many report that writing the methods section is "easy" because these are the core facts of how the work was completed. However, writing methods description is more challenging if you have not taken good notes along the way.

- Results: This section is written to summarize what you found. This is definitely something you write later, after all the data are collected and analyzed. Think objectively about the results section and simply report what you found without a great deal of interpretation. You will save your interpretations for the discussion section.

- Discussion: You will use this section to discuss the work and your interpretations of the results. It's expected that you will write something that goes beyond a simple analysis of the data alone. What do your results mean? How should they be interpreted? How do they relate or connect to what the previous literature reported? What cautions should the reader take when interpreting your findings? This can lead you to a direct and clear discussion about the *limitations* of your work. Remember, limitations aren't necessarily a deadly thing, just something you need to acknowledge. Discussion sections can take significant thought and conversation. If you have presented your work as a presentation or poster (see Chapter 11) before writing a manuscript, you may have interacted with people who have helped shape your thinking of the discussion. These conversations are gifts to you, and you should note them along the way so that you can incorporate them into your work. Both authors of this chapter have taken some excellent notes during presentations where we have learned a great deal from our colleagues! It can shape your discussion section, and your work.

- Future Directions: This can be a fun section to write. What's next? Where are the future areas of study? How do any strengths or challenges of your own work influence future research questions? What are the next burning issues? Many times, you can find a great deal of inspiration here.

This broad outline gives you a start and helps you to consider how you might begin putting your thoughts together for a peer-reviewed journal article. However, this outline isn't the only place you should be looking. You'll also want to read the directions laid out for you in any "Instructions to Authors/Submissions" page at the website of the journal where you might be publishing. Often, starting with this outline gives you something to work with and adapt as you move along.

## Manuscript Preparation Details

Submitting your work for publication will vary from venue to venue. The journal's web pages will have some content, often labeled "Author Guidelines" that will detail how to format your manuscript for submission. It is critical that you consult and follow these guidelines carefully. However, there are some general things to consider:

- There will likely be limits on the number of pages you are allowed to submit.
- Submissions will likely be double-spaced with 11- or 12-point and using standard fonts (e.g., Arial, Times New Roman). It is possible you will need to use your word processing program to number the lines of your manuscript for easy reference.
- Manuscript wording should be formal rather than informal. Use an active voice whenever possible. Spell out acronyms prior to abbreviating them and define terms that may not be familiar to your target audience. Avoid contractions, colloquialisms, and self-referencing (unless it is critical to your positionality as a researcher).
- Tables and figures will typically be submitted as separate, individual files. Therefore, don't spend a great deal of time trying to embed them into a document. Instead, you will reference where the tables and figures should be inserted in the document using statements like "Place Figure 1 about here." It can be a real time saver to not need to focus on embedding tables and figures into a document!
- Pay meticulous attention to your references along the way. This can avoid hours of last-minute frustrating cross-checks. The last step in submitting your original or revised manuscript should be to ensure that every reference in your reference list appears in your text and that every reference that appears in the text is also included in the reference list.

- Note that we discussed copyright in this chapter. Depending on the journal's copyright policy, you may not be able to simply "borrow" tables or figures from other authors. Instead, you will either need to adapt them or seek permission to publish them from the original publisher. This may take time. Follow the directions of your publisher closely knowing that these permissions are not always granted quickly or easily. If you see a notation regarding the use of "Creative Commons" in the journal's information about copyright, that may mean that you can use the information without written permission as long as you attribute the original source accurately. If you are in doubt, search the specific type of Creative Commons listed on the internet.
- When in doubt? For most fields, following the *Publication Manual of the American Psychological Association, Seventh Edition* (2020) can be a safe start. Consult the journal's web page to see if they have a style guide that they default to. It will be important to comply with their expectations.

---

### Box 12-7:
### Plagiarism

Most clinicians have had education in avoiding plagiarism throughout their academic careers. We want to remind you that plagiarism is serious. It is possible that a code of ethics for a professional association has language about adequately citing and quoting the work of others. We would like you to think even one layer deeper as a clinician engaging in research, however. At what point might you plagiarize yourself? Self-plagiarism is a real concern. Self-plagiarism might mean you "recycle" elements of your work (or large pieces of it, for that matter) without attributing it appropriately. It might be tempting to think, "I'm writing something similar to some of my past work, so I will start by editing my previous work." *We do not advise this.* Instead, read your previous work like you would any other publication you might reference. Then, reference your work appropriately by starting "fresh" with any new publication.

---

## A Word About Article Types and Journals

Even in a peer-reviewed, also known as refereed, journal, not all articles are peer reviewed. For instance, editorials and book reviews (although solicited by the journal) do not undergo the same review process.

## Box 12-8:
## Predatory Journals

Some journals require a fee for publication of your article. This may occur even if your manuscript has undergone a peer-review process. Other journals demand a fee for publication in lieu of the review process. Beware! These journals are termed "predatory" and should be avoided at all costs. A predatory journal is only self-serving; odds are it will publish findings without a significant review or editorial changes. Predatory journals are seen as a detriment to the scientific method and dissemination of valid results. A recent consensus definition for these journals was cited as, "Predatory journals and publishers are entities that prioritize self-interest at the expense of scholarship and are characterized by false or misleading information, deviation from best editorial and publication practices, a lack of transparency, and/or the use of aggressive and indiscriminate solicitation practices" (Grudniewicz et al., 2019). Recognize that there are more than 10,000 journals deemed predatory; be suspicious if your work is solicited without your query to a journal—it is likely a predatory journal. Always investigate the editorial board of any journal you are thinking of submitting your work to, as this will confirm that the editors have expertise in your field of study.

To determine if a journal is peer reviewed, limit your database search of journals in your field to those that are peer reviewed. If a member of your team is affiliated with a university library, searches of Scopus or Web of Science will lead you to refereed journals in your field of expertise. You may also go directly to a journal's website and look at the "Submissions" tab. The process of submission will be discussed here and allow you to see if the journal requires the peer-review process.

## Last Steps in the Process

At this point, you have some ideas about the process for publication. You can see that there is much to consider! There are a few more things you should know about, regardless of where you elect to publish your work. These things will be driven by timelines and should not be ignored.

- You will need to revise your manuscript based on editor/reviewer feedback. Note that when you receive this feedback, you will be given a timeline for making any changes.
- Once all changes are complete and accepted, the editor will "accept" your manuscript. This is a great feeling—but you aren't done! The editor will likely inform you of a publication timeline and you'll be notified about "proofs" coming your way.

- A copyeditor will engage with your manuscript and make small editorial changes and work to have the manuscript put in its final layout or form for the publication type. The copyeditor may have a few questions for you, so you should be watching for communications along the way.
- Proofs (sometimes called "page proofs" or "galley proofs") will be your final stop. Proofs will be your opportunity to see how the manuscript will appear on the page for the reader. Note: Proofs are a point where you can make final and critical changes. However, this point is *not* an opportunity for you to start rewriting your work. Instead, you should be looking for any very small changes that are critical to the message of your work.
- Get ready to see your work in print! Once you have approved your proofs and understand the timeline for moving the work to your audience, you might want to consider letting your audience know through any presentations you may have scheduled and your professional social media accounts.

## Box 12-9:
## Take Your Time With Proofs/Copyedits

Take focused time and energy with proofs. This is your last stop along the way. Something small, like forgetting the word "not," could dramatically change your intended message. You should take your time with proofs and read and reread. Having an additional set of eyes can be useful in this process as well. Here is where your board of mentors could be of additional assistance.

## Acknowledging Your Work on Your Curriculum Vitae

As you go through the paper submission process, it may be reflected on your professional curriculum vitae (CV). A manuscript submitted to a journal may be listed on your professional CV as "submitted for review," along with the journal name prior to its acceptance. If the manuscript is selected to undergo review, you may change this on your CV to reflect "under review." Finally, if your manuscript is accepted for publication, you may indicate this on your CV as "accepted." When you are given specifics about the publication date, the issue, page numbers, and so on, you will change your CV to reflect the publication.

If your work is not going to be peer reviewed, you might consider developing different categories on your CV, depending upon what is conventional in your discipline. For instance, you might have categories such as:

- Peer-reviewed works
- Books and book chapters
- State- and regional-level publications

If you are engaging with a blog, you might direct a reviewer of your CV to it right in your identifying information on the CV.

# A Word About Authorship

Much of what you have been reading in this text makes it appear that you will be working on your research alone. We know this is entirely unrealistic and impractical. You'll likely engage with a team of other people (your board of mentors?) to put your work together and get it published. Major challenges can arise if you have not considered—and openly discussed— potential authorship of the work at the beginning and again along the way. Who will be authors? Are there people who contributed but aren't necessarily authors of the work? Do they understand their role? Who is the first author? What is conventional for your discipline in terms of the order of authorship? For many, a "first author" role means greatest ownership of the research and writing. However, you will want to look for and understand what is conventional in your field (e.g., it is possible that the last author listed is indicative of significant contribution). Why should you have these conversations early? You want to avoid conflict and challenges to the publication process right up front. A good practice is to meet, agree, and send minutes to all parties of what you have agreed upon in terms of authorship with an acknowledgment from each person. This is all part of beginning with the end in mind!

## Box 12-10:
### Acknowledgments

Acknowledgments are a way for you to recognize someone who is a significant contributor to your work, yet not an author. For instance, you might acknowledge a statistician, a mentor, specific students, or even a group who has funded your work. However, academic journals do not typically offer an opportunity for acknowledging those who have offered emotional or moral support.

# Reflection and Planning

Now, step back to that original reflection you had at the beginning of the chapter. You took a few moments to dream and consider where your work might be published. However, you did that without the information in this chapter. Head back to your original thoughts and notes. Have things changed? Do you have realistic expectations for where your work might be published? Are you considering the advice from a trusted mentor who has previously published their work? Are they on board with contributing to your future? You now have some basic tools to put you at the ready for a conversation about your best hopes—as well as a backup plan.

## Backup Plans for Publishing

You might receive a variety of advice about publishing your work and considering backup plans. Some might advise you, "Make a plan and stick with it. Tell yourself you won't fail." We appreciate that enthusiasm entirely and encourage you to believe in yourself and your hard work. However, we also hold true to having a backup plan as well.

Why a backup plan? This helps you avoid making a failure-based decision in the future. We are not advising you to overthink the backup plan. Instead, consider, "We are submitting our work to [insert name of first-choice journal]. We'll keep presenting our work and listen to feedback while the manuscript is under review. If it isn't a fit for our first-choice journal, our next step will be to submit it to [insert name of journal here]." This means you have a plan, and you aren't in a scramble should your work be rejected by your first choice.

What's within the backup plan? Something nested within a backup plan is the gift of feedback. If your first submission is rejected, you'll have reviewer feedback and you'll understand why a negative decision was made regarding the work. This will give you an opportunity to retool the manuscript before you submit it to another journal. Although negative feedback can feel punishing, it can make for an excellent product in the end.

Don't delay! Start thinking about your dissemination plan—and your backup plan—today!

# REFERENCES

American Psychological Association. (2020). *Publication manual of the American Psychological Association 2020: The official guide to APA style* (7th ed.). Author.

Bernstein, J. L. (2011). Reviewer essay: Identifying high quality SoTL research: A perspective from a reviewer. *International Journal for the Scholarship of Teaching and Learning, 5*(1), article 37. https://doi.org/10.20429/ijsotl.2011.050137

Covey, S. (1989). *The seven habits of highly effective people.* Simon & Schuster.

Grudniewicz, A., Moher, D., Cobey, K. D., Bryson, G. L., Cukier, S., Allen, K., Ardern, C., Balcom, L., Barros, T., Berger, M., Ciro, J. B., Cugusi, L., Donaldson, M. R., Egger, M., Graham, I. D., Hodgkinson, M., Khan, K. M., Mabizela, M., Manca, A., … Lalu, M. M. (2019). Predatory journals: No definition, no defense. *Nature, 576*(7786), 210-212. Springer Science and Business Media LLC. https://doi.org/10.1038/d41586-019-03759-y

Quinn, C. T., & Rush, A. J. (2009). Writing and publishing your research findings. *Journal of Investigative Medicine: The Official Publication of the American Federation for Clinical Research, 57*(5), 634-639. https://doi.org/10.2310/JIM.0b013e3181a39164

# Worksheet 12-1:
# Publishing Your Research

What is the focus of your research publication?

| |
|---|
| |

Who is your audience?

| |
|---|
| |

**Publication Venues**

| Book/Chapter/Blog | Journal (Profession vs. SoTL?) |
|---|---|
| Plan A: | Plan A: |
| Plan B: | Plan B: |

**Manuscript Outline**

- Title
- Abstract
- Introduction
- Research question
- Hypothesis (quantitative research only)
- Methods
- Results
- Discussion
  - Limitations
- Future directions

Publication strategies: What is the best way to get your work to your target audience? ("Safe" vs. "Top Tier")

| |
|---|
| |

# FINANCIAL DISCLOSURES

*Dr. Jessica Brown* reported no financial or proprietary interest in the materials presented herein.

*Jordan Dann* reported no financial or proprietary interest in the materials presented herein.

*Dr. Mark DeRuiter* reported no financial or proprietary interest in the materials presented herein.

*Dr. Carol C. Dudding* reported no financial or proprietary interest in the materials presented herein.

*Dr. Lizbeth H. Finestack* reported no financial or proprietary interest in the materials presented herein.

*Dr. Sarah M. Ginsberg* reported no financial or proprietary interest in the materials presented herein.

*Dr. Elizabeth A. VandeWaa* reported no financial or proprietary interest in the materials presented herein.

*Dr. Patrick R. Walden* reported no financial or proprietary interest in the materials presented herein.

*Dr. Jayne Yatczak* reported no financial or proprietary interest in the materials presented herein.

# Index

Printed in the United States
by Baker & Taylor Publisher Services